Free Tissue Transfer to Head and Neck: Lessons Learned from Unfavorable Results

Editors

FU-CHAN WEI
NIDAL FARHAN AL DEEK

CLINICS IN PLASTIC SURGERY

www.plasticsurgery.theclinics.com

October 2016 • Volume 43 • Number 4

ELSEVIER

1600 John F. Kennedy Boulevard ● Suite 1800 ● Philadelphia, Pennsylvania, 19103-2899

http://www.theclinics.com

CLINICS IN PLASTIC SURGERY Volume 43, Number 4
October 2016 ISSN 0094-1298, ISBN-13: 978-0-323-46331-7

Editor: Jessica McCool
Developmental Editor: Donald Mumford

Clinics in Plastic Surgery (ISSN 0094-1298) is published quarterly by Elsevier Inc., 360 Park Avenue South, New York, NY 10010-1710. Months of issue are January, April, July, and October. Business and Editorial Offices: 1600 John F. Kennedy Blvd., Suite 1800, Philadelphia, PA 19103-2899. Periodicals postage paid at New York, NY and additional mailing offices. Subscription prices are $490.00 per year for US individuals, $793.00 per year for US institutions, $100.00 per year for US students and residents, $555.00 per year for Canadian individuals, $944.00 per year for Canadian institutions, $630.00 per year for international individuals, $944.00 per year for international institutions, and $305.00 per year for Canadian and foreign students/residents. To receive student/resident rate, orders must be accompanied by name of affiliated institution, date of term, and the *signature* of program/residency coordinator on institution letterhead. Orders will be billed at individual rate until proof of status is received. Foreign air speed delivery is included in all *Clinics* subscription prices. All prices are subject to change without notice. **POSTMASTER:** Send address changes to *Clinics in Plastic Surgery*, Elsevier Health Sciences Division, Subscription Customer Service, 3251 Riverport Lane, Maryland Heights, MO 63043. **Customer Service: 1-800-654-2452 (US and Canada). From outside of the United States and Canada, call 314-447-8871. Fax: 314-447-8029. E-mail: JournalsCustomerService-usa@elsevier.com (for print support); JournalsOnlineSupport-usa@ elsevier.com (for online support).**

Reprints. For copies of 100 or more of articles in this publication, please contact the Commercial Reprints Department, Elsevier Inc., 360 Park Avenue South, New York, New York 10010-1710. Tel.: +1-212-633-3874; Fax: +1-212-633-3820; E-mail: reprints@elsevier.com.

Clinics in Plastic Surgery is covered in *Current Contents, EMBASE/Excerpta Medica, Science Citation Index, MEDLINE/ PubMed (Index Medicus), ASCA,* and *ISI/BIOMED.*

Contributors

EDITORS

FU-CHAN WEI, MD, FACS
Distinguished Chair Professor, Department of
Plastic and Reconstructive Surgery, Chang
Gung Memorial Hospital, Chang Gung
University Medical College, Chang Gung
University, Taipei, Taiwan

NIDAL FARHAN AL DEEK, MSc, MD
Department of Plastic and Reconstructive
Surgery, Chang Gung Memorial Hospital,
Chang Gung Medical College, Chang Gung
University, Taipei, Taiwan

AUTHORS

NIDAL FARHAN AL DEEK, MSc, MD
Department of Plastic and Reconstructive
Surgery, Chang Gung Memorial Hospital,
Chang Gung Medical College, Chang Gung
University, Taipei, Taiwan

SCOTT E. BEVANS, MD
Clinical Instructor, Department of
Otolaryngology, University of Washington,
Seattle, Washington

ROMAIN BOSC, MD
Service de Chirurgie Plastique,
Reconstructrice, Esthétique et Maxillofaciale,
Henri Mondor Hospital, Créteil, France

JAMES BROWN, MD, FRCS, FDSRCS
Consultant and Honorary Professor,
Department of Head and Neck Surgery, Aintree
University Hospital; Northwest Cancer
Research Centre, Liverpool University,
Liverpool, United Kingdom

CHARLES E. BUTLER, MD
Professor and Chair, Department of Plastic
Surgery, The University of Texas MD Anderson
Cancer Center, Houston, Texas

**CHRIS BUTTERWORTH, BDS(Hons), MPhil,
FDSRCS, FDS(Rest), RCS(Eng)**
Consultant and Honorary Senior Lecturer,
Maxillofacial Prosthodontics, Aintree University
Hospital; Prosthodontic Department, Liverpool
University Dental Hospital, Liverpool, United
Kingdom

EDWARD I. CHANG, MD
Assistant Professor, Department of Plastic
Surgery, The University of Texas MD Anderson
Cancer Center, Houston, Texas

YANG-MING CHANG, DDS
Department of Plastic and Reconstructive
Surgery, Chang Gung Memorial Hospital,
Chang Gung Medical College, Chang Gung
University, Taipei, Taiwan

MING-HUEI CHENG, MD, MBA, FACS
Department of Plastic and Reconstructive
Surgery, Chang Gung Memorial Hospital,
Chang Gung Medical College, Chang Gung
University, Taipei, Taiwan

ERIKA DE LA CONCHA, MD
Department of Plastic and Reconstructive
Surgery, Hospital General Dr. Manuel Gea
Gonzalez, Mexico City, Mexico

NEAL D. FUTRAN, MD
Professor, Department of Otolaryngology,
University of Washington, Seattle, Washington

MATTHEW M. HANASONO, MD
Professor, Department of Plastic Surgery,
The University of Texas MD Anderson Cancer
Center, Houston, Texas

RICHARD E. HAYDEN, MD
Professor, Department of Otolaryngology-Head
and Neck Surgery, Mayo Clinic, Phoenix,
Arizona

STEFAN O.P. HOFER, MD, PhD, FRCSC
Full Professor of Surgery; Wharton Chair in
Head and Neck Reconstruction; Head,
Division of Plastic Surgery, Department of
Surgery, University Health Network,
University of Toronto, Toronto, Ontario,
Canada

JEFFREY J. HOULTON, MD
Assistant Professor, Department of
Otolaryngology, University of Washington,
Seattle, Washington

HUANG-KAI KAO, MD
Department of Plastic and Reconstructive
Surgery, Chang Gung Memorial Hospital,
Chang Gung Medical College, Chang Gung
University, Taipei, Taiwan

YOSHIHIRO KIMATA, MD
Professor and Chairman, Department of
Plastic and Reconstructive Surgery, Okayama
University, Graduate School of Medicine,
Dentistry and Pharmaceutical Sciences,
Okayama University, Okayama City,
Okayama, Japan

MARIKA KUUSKERI, MD, PhD
Clinical Fellow, Reconstructive Microsurgery,
Division of Plastic Surgery, Department of
Surgery, University Health Network, University
of Toronto, Toronto, Ontario, Canada

ILYA LIKHTEROV, MD
Assistant Professor, Head and Neck
Oncologic and Reconstructive Surgery,
Department of Otolaryngology, Mount Sinai
Beth Israel, New York, New York

CHIH-HUNG LIN, MD
Department of Plastic and Reconstructive
Surgery, Chang Gung Memorial Hospital,
Chang Gung Medical College, Chang Gung
University, Taipei, Taiwan

HIROSHI MATSUMOTO, MD
Assistant Professor, Department of Plastic
and Reconstructive Surgery, Okayama
University, Graduate School of Medicine,
Dentistry and Pharmaceutical Sciences,
Okayama University, Okayama City, Okayama,
Japan

JEAN-PAUL MENINGAUD, MD, PhD
Service de Chirurgie Plastique,
Reconstructrice, Esthétique et
Maxillofaciale, Henri Mondor Hospital,
Créteil, France

THOMAS H. NAGEL, MD
Assistant Professor, Department of
Otolaryngology-Head and Neck Surgery,
Mayo Clinic, Phoenix, Arizona

**ANNE C. O'NEILL, MBBCh, MMedSci,
FRCS(Plast), MSc, PhD**
Assistant Professor, Division of Plastic
Surgery, Department of Surgery, University
Health Network, University of Toronto,
Toronto, Ontario, Canada

SATOSHI ONODA, MD
Assistant Professor, Department of Plastic
and Reconstructive Surgery, Okayama
University, Graduate School of Medicine,
Dentistry and Pharmaceutical Sciences,
Okayama University, Okayama City,
Okayama, Japan

MINORU SAKURABA, MD
Head, Division of Head and Neck Surgery,
National Cancer Center Hospital East,
Kashiwa, Chiba, Japan

ERIC SANTAMARIA, MD
Associate Professor, Department of
Plastic and Reconstructive Surgery;
Head of Microsurgery Clinic, Hospital
General Dr. Manuel Gea Gonzalez,
National Cancer Institute, Universidad
Nacional Autonoma de Mexico,
Mexico City, Mexico

**ANDREW SCHACHE, PhD, FRCS,
FDSRCS**
Consultant and Senior Lecturer,
Department of Head and Neck Surgery,
Aintree University Hospital; Northwest
Cancer Research Centre, Liverpool
University, Liverpool,
United Kingdom

NARUSI SUGIYAMA, MD
Assistant Professor, Department of Plastic
and Reconstructive Surgery, Okayama
University, Graduate School of Medicine,
Dentistry and Pharmaceutical Sciences,
Okayama University, Okayama City, Okayama,
Japan

CHUNG-KAN TSAO, MD
Department of Plastic and Reconstructive
Surgery, Chang Gung Memorial Hospital,
Chang Gung Medical College, Chang Gung
University, Taipei, Taiwan

MARK URKEN, MD, FACS, FACE
Chief, Division of Head and Neck Surgical
Oncology, Department of Otolaryngology,
Mount Sinai Beth Israel, New York,
New York

FU-CHAN WEI, MD, FACS
Distinguished Chair Professor,
Department of Plastic and Reconstructive
Surgery, Chang Gung Memorial Hospital,
Chang Gung University Medical College,
Chang Gung University, Taipei,
Taiwan

Contents

The Triangle of Unfavorable Outcomes After Microsurgical Head and Neck Reconstruction: Planning, Design, and Execution 615

Fu-Chan Wei, Nidal Farhan AL Deek, Ming-Huei Cheng, and Chih-Hung Lin

Analysis of unfavorable results in microsurgical head and neck reconstruction beyond free flap survival is the goal of this article. Unfavorable outcome is the result of poor or inadequate planning, design, and execution. A triangular relationship between the 3 corners of a microsurgical reconstruction—plan, design, and execution—is suggested to govern the unfavorable outcome after a surviving free flap. This article shares the authors' philosophy and strategies to avoid untoward outcomes. Case studies and the authors' surgery dynamics are provided to simplify the message.

Free Tissue Transfer to Head and Neck: Lessons Learned from Unfavorable Results—Experience per Subsite 621

Nidal Farhan AL Deek, Fu-Chan Wei, and Huang-Kai Kao

This article provides a lesson-learned approach per site and anatomic structure to head and neck reconstruction. It addresses the most common unfavorable results following successful free flap transfer, shedding light on why they happen and how to prevent them. It draws from hundreds of advanced and complicated microsurgical head and neck reconstruction cases, aiming to achieve excellence in the reconstructive endeavor and to enhance the patient's quality of life.

Mount Sinai Medical Center and Their Experience with Unfavorable Microsurgical Head and Neck Reconstruction 631

Ilya Likhterov and Mark Urken

Radiation effects on tissues greatly complicate reconstruction of head and neck defects. We discuss the unfavorable surgical conditions set up by prior surgery and radiation in patients undergoing salvage ablation of recurrent cancer. With the focus on vessel selection, flap donor site characteristics, and management of potential complications, we hope to highlight some of the lessons learned from these complex cases. Special attention is given to the topic of laryngopharyngeal reconstruction.

Unfavorable Results After Free Tissue Transfer to Head and Neck: Lessons Based on Experience from the University of Toronto 639

Marika Kuuskeri, Anne C. O'Neill, and Stefan O.P. Hofer

The purpose of the current article is to provide an overview of the functional and aesthetic unfavorable results of head and neck reconstruction, and provide suggestions on how to address these issues. Understanding the consequences of an unsuccessful reconstruction provides the foundation for proper planning and personalized approach to reconstruction of lost structures.

This article addresses trismus following head and neck cancer ablation and free flap reconstruction whether or not radiotherapy has been utilized. The focus is to achieve durable and favorable outcomes and avoid untoward results. To aid surgeons in fulfilling these goals, key factors, including adequate release surgery, optimal free flap selection and reconstruction, long-lasting results, and the untoward outcomes specific to trismus release and reconstruction surgery and how to avoid them have been investigated and discussed based on the authors' experience in this surgery.

Osteoradionecrosis is preferably called osteosarcoradionecrosis to adequately cover the scope of the problem: multitissue necrosis. The changes following radiotherapy and leading to necrosis are further classified into 2 phases based on improved understanding of the underlying mechanisms. The reversible-damage phase could respond to the medical treatment, while the irreversible damage phase or osteosarcoradionecrosis may benefit from complete resection and free flap reconstruction. The role of ablation and reconstruction in paving the road for the development of osteosarcoradionecrosis is discussed, a case study provided, and a refined reconstructive approach proposed.

CLINICS IN PLASTIC SURGERY

THE CLINICS ARE AVAILABLE ONLINE!
Access your subscription at:
www.theclinics.com

Preface
The Unfavorable Outcome: Here We Conquer

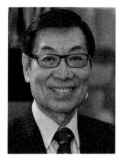
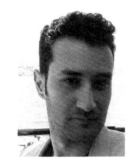

Fu-Chan Wei, MD, FACS   Nidal Farhan AL Deek, MSc, MD

Editors

Microsurgical reconstruction of the head and neck defects is the gold standard of treatment. Success rates are in the region of 98% in most of the major referral centers. Traditionally, success is defined by the patency of microvascular anastomosis and free flap viability. However, as we grow more critical about our success, its definition has evolved to refer to the successful restoration of function and appearance with improved patient quality of life.

Achieving a successful reconstruction beyond flap survival is, therefore, a challenging, experience-demanding endeavor that necessitates a comprehensive understanding of the unfavorable outcomes. This includes why and how they happen as well as strategies to avoid and manage them.

Information on the unfavorable outcomes after a microsurgical head and neck reconstruction gone wrong despite successful free flap surgery is lacking. The paucity of information in the literature is the impetus for this special issue of *Clinics in Plastic Surgery*. Our aim is to provide an immense, experience-based reflection with sincere accounts from the experts on the unfavorable outcomes after microsurgical reconstruction of the head and neck. And, our hope is that this work will help guide surgeons to achieve success in restoring human dignity with good function and aesthetics.

The content is organized into three subcategories, including (1) the unfavorable outcomes in microsurgical head and neck reconstruction: what they are and why they happen; (2) specific discussion on the unfavorable outcomes per subsite, empowered by case-based illustrations to educate on the untoward outcomes or demonstrate how international experts in world-renowned centers approach these problems; and (3) avoidance and management of specific unfavorable results commonly seen in microsurgical head and neck reconstruction.

We are very proud to say that each of the authors is an authority in head and neck microsurgical reconstruction. This issue is a fusion of knowledge gained from years of experience in a wealth of varying disciplines such as head and neck surgery, maxillofacial surgery, and plastic surgery.

We would specifically like to extend our sincerest gratitude to them for making this a highlight issue of the prestigious and renowned series *Clinics in Plastic Surgery*.

We also would like to thank the team from Elsevier for their great effort and kind assistance in making this work a reality. In particular, we would like to thank Jessica McCool and Don Mumford for their support and help; it was a great pleasure working with them.

We sincerely hope that you, the reader, will find this issue useful in planning the reconstruction in

Clin Plastic Surg 43 (2016) xiii–xiv
http://dx.doi.org/10.1016/j.cps.2016.08.001
0094-1298/16/© 2016 Published by Elsevier Inc.

such a way that results in fewer complications and enhances your patient quality of life.

Fu-Chan Wei, MD, FACS
Department of Plastic and Reconstructive Surgery
Chang Gung Memorial Hospital
Chang Gung Medical College
Chang Gung University
199 Tun-Hwa North Road
Taipei 10591, Taiwan

Nidal Farhan AL Deek, MSc, MD
Department of Plastic and Reconstructive Surgery
Chang Gung Memorial Hospital
Chang Gung Medical College
Chang Gung University
199 Tun-Hwa North Road
Taipei 10591, Taiwan

E-mail addresses:
fuchanwei@gmail.com (F.-C. Wei)
nidaldeek@gmail.com (N.F. AL Deek)

The Triangle of Unfavorable Outcomes After Microsurgical Head and Neck Reconstruction
Planning, Design, and Execution

Fu-Chan Wei, MD*, Nidal Farhan AL Deek, MSc, MD,
Ming-Huei Cheng, MD, MBA, Chih-Hung Lin, MD

KEYWORDS

- Head and neck reconstruction • Microsurgical reconstruction • Quality of life • Unfavorable results
- Failure

KEY POINTS

- Unfavorable microsurgical reconstruction, independent from free flap failure, is an important concept; understanding and avoidance of the unfavorable outcome enhances patient's quality of life.
- Unfavorable microsurgical reconstruction is the result of defective planning and decision making, inapt design, and faulty execution in a triangular interrelationship.
- Inexperience, inadequate discussion, vague goals, ineffective communication, and lack of sincere reflection on untoward outcomes pave the roads for adversities in reconstruction.

INTRODUCTION

For a long time, the outcomes of microsurgical head and neck reconstruction have been reported in the form of free flap survival rate, disease-free survival rate, and 5-year survival rate, reflecting what mattered at the time: achieving reliability of the techniques used in ablation and reconstruction surgeries. But, reliability of microsurgical techniques nowadays along with improved survival rates after advanced head and neck tumor ablation and the rising need for additional surgeries to treat reconstruction sequelae to improve function or appearance[1–5] have brought about the importance of considering a patient's quality of life.[6,7]

Thinking of a patient's quality of life leads to defining success and failure of reconstruction differently. Success refers not only to survival of a flap but also to adequately restoring function and appearance to ensure good patient living after surgery as expected. Failure refers to inadequately achieving that goal despite flap survival. Failure can be marked by prolonged hospitalization, readmissions, or secondary surgeries, to achieve what has been failed to gain the first time.

Herein, avoidance of failure in achieving the reconstructive goals that a viable flap should serve is of paramount importance to the core theme of contemporary microsurgical head and neck reconstruction.

An unfavorable result can arise from an error in any of the 3 major phases of the reconstructive microsurgery. Defective planning and decision making is 1 faulty scenario. Inapt design and

Conflict of Interest: The authors have no conflict of interest to declare.
Department of Plastic and Reconstructive Surgery, Chang Gung Memorial Hospital, Chang Gung Medical College, Chang Gung University, 199 Tun-Hwa North Road, Taipei 10591, Taiwan
* Corresponding author.
E-mail address: fuchanwei@gmail.com

Clin Plastic Surg 43 (2016) 615–620
http://dx.doi.org/10.1016/j.cps.2016.06.001

erroneous reconstruction are other possibilities. However, an unfavorable result is the bitter fruit of failing to a variable degree in all of these 3 aspects, suggesting an independent yet closely related interactive triangle in which every corner/angle can lead to unfavorable outcome alone or by contributing to a collective effect of the triangle (**Fig. 1**).

There are still many variables, however, in head and neck reconstruction that cannot be controlled, or predicted, such as spontaneous and radiation-induced tissue atrophy, fibrosis plate exposure, wound contracture, and possible osteoradionecrosis.[8,9] Striving to bestow the best quality of life possible on patients imposes a responsibility to always explore the underlying causes behind an unfavorable result and to take into consideration the variables (discussed previously) to pioneer a technique and/or refine another to minimize the negative impact of those variables on the quality of reconstruction and enhance the outcome.

THE TRIANGLE OF UNFAVORABLE OUTCOMES
Defective Planning and Decision Making

Definition
Defective planning and decision making refers to an error in the reconstructive approach, such as 1-stage versus staged and optimal versus suboptimal, or the extent of the reconstructive endeavor, for instance, to address the defect only versus the defect and the underlying conditions, such as trismus, fibrosis, and so forth. It also refers to error

in the selection of the flap, perforator/skin vessel, and recipient vessels.

After deciding on a microsurgical reconstruction, the planning should address the following.

Should it be a 1-stage total reconstruction or staged reconstruction?
This is a key question addressing, for example, mandibular and maxillary defects.

The right answer should take into account prognosis, anticipated defect characteristics, realistic patient's goals, and expected postoperative course. Based on these, the answer or the plan can be thorough and governs flap selection, bony versus soft tissue flap, and the number of flaps needed as well as the demand for subsequent touch-up procedures, such as sensory restoration after inferior alveolar nerve resection, immediate or delayed dental rehabilitation in mandibular reconstruction, and so forth.[10]

What are the priority goals of reconstruction, and how can he chosen flap(s) be used to fulfill these goals?
Head and neck defects can be extensive, spanning multiple subsites, or involve sophisticated structures, such as the tongue, the lips, the eye, and so forth. Autologous tissue is limited and in many occasions cannot replace the lost delicate structures, especially at the same time. Prioritizing the reconstruction, therefore, is essential to fulfill a patient's goal and minimize dissatisfaction or complications.

Planning is also concerned with achieving and maintaining good results, for example, how to achieve good occlusion and trismus-free reconstruction, prevent tissue sagging, and so forth. Also, surgeons should remind themselves in planning with the important need for certain surgical procedures not related to free flap surgery itself, such as preplating, intraoperative navigation, coronoidotomy, suspension, and so forth, to allow enough time for preparation and effective utilization in the surgery.

Last but not least, planning should address free tissue donor sites. Although many flaps can do the work, only few have the advantages of 2-team approach and versatile design, especially after previous microsurgical reconstructions. Taking versatility, ergonomics and logistics, and donor site morbidity into account, flaps from lower extremity, in particular, the anterolateral thigh (ALT) flap and the fibula osteoseptocutaneous flap, have taken over head and neck reconstruction, signaling a decline in using other donor sites.[11–13]

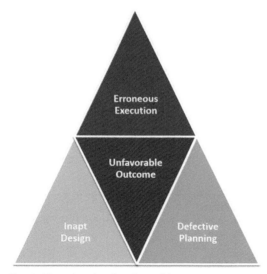

Fig. 1. The triangle of unfavorable outcome.

Case 1: defective planning

A 61-year-old male patient, whose history was significant for left lower gum squamous cell carcinoma, T4aN0M0, for which he received compound segmental mandibulectomy and fibula osteoseptocutaneous flap reconstruction, in 2006 presented with recurrent squamous cell carcinoma; rT2N0M0, at the left lower gum, in 2009. Tumor ablation necessitated composite segmental mandibulectomy with resection of the previous fibula flap. Ablation succeeded in increasing mouth opening to 20 mm. The defect involved segmental mandibulectomy from midline to angle, 8 × 8 cm mucosal defect and 7 × 6 cm skin defect.

Because of the patient's limited mouth opening initially and anticipated poor prognosis, a staged mandibular reconstruction was thought acceptable, and a reconstruction plate with composite myocutaneous ALT flap was used.

The patient, however, had a good life span but suffered from malocclusion, plate fracture, trismus, and Andy Gump deformity (**Fig. 2**).

Defective planning is usually the result of inadequate discussion and analysis of the anticipated problem(s) with poor communication among the team members. It is important, thus, to harness the planning prowess to determine the reconstructive attitude and the amount of reconstructive effort to be invested in a given case, prioritize the reconstruction goals, remain steadfast in fulfilling them, and provide a list of techniques to be used so that all team members remain on the same page.

All of that is done in a way connecting the present with the future of the patient and the current defect with years from the time of actual surgery.

Inapt Design

Definition

Inapt design refers to a mistake in designing flap shape and orientation, tissue component(s) transferred with the flap, or the inter-relationship between any of these components, leading to failure in achieving optimal results. The concept can also be extended to address plates, templates, and cutting guides used in isolated, compound, and composite bony reconstruction.

The ALT flap, a workhorse flap, can be used to further explain the importance of design. Where to design the flap on the thigh, for example, to carry a thicker tissue or thinner tissue has a toll on the quality of oral reconstruction and the need for additional flap thinning; similarly is the level of dissection: below the fascia, above the fascia, and above the Scarpa fascia.[12,14]

The inter-relationship between flap components, which is experience-demanding, should be carefully designed to best fulfill the reconstruction goals and to allow the reconstruction to be flexible and dynamic.

Myocutaneous flaps can illustrate the importance of good intercomponent design. There are 2 types of myocutaneous flaps to be used depending on skin-muscle inter-relationship. In a combined design, both the muscle and skin have

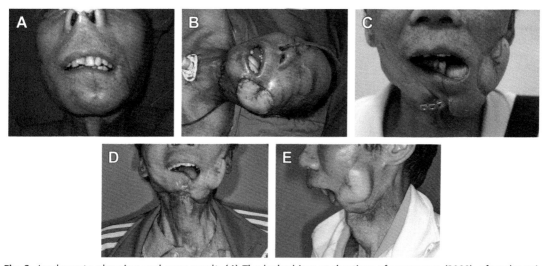

Fig. 2. Inadequate planning and poor result. (*A*) The locked jaw at the time of recurrence (2009), after the primary gum cancer was treated with segmental mandibulectomy and fibula reconstruction followed by radiotherapy in 2006. (*B*) The composite mandibulectomy defect after excision of recurrent cancer was treated with a reconstruction palate and a huge ALT myocutaneous flap without bone. (*C*) Exposure and fracture of reconstruction plate. (*D, E*) Andy Gump deformity after removal of reconstruction plate.

independent blood supply yet are joined together by a common source pedicle.[15,16] This design is suitable for complex 3-D configuration and multi-subsite reconstruction. In a composite myocutaneous flap design, tissues are dependent on each other for supply.[15,16] This design may not be able to address defects of complex 3-D configuration and involve multisubsites adequately without compromising the flap circulation, which may cause flap necrosis, wound dehiscence, or fistula formation.

Templates and cutting guides are useful during bone osteotomy and contouring. Poorly designed templates may result in bony segments of inappropriate length or imperfect contact surface between the bony struts compromising union.

Case 2: inapt design

A 74-year-old male patient presented with right soft palate squamous cell carcinoma, T1N0M0; 50% of the soft palate was resected. Reconstruction was achieved by fasciocutaneous ALT flap measuring 22 × 8 cm.

The flap used was thick and large; therefore, it resulted in compromised soft palate function and airway compression with prolonged intubation; subsequent revisions were necessary to improve function and appearance. A smaller and thinner flap should have been used (**Fig. 3**).

Good flap design is thus important to achieve favorable function and appearance. This step is better done by the experienced surgeon of the team. Avoidance of inapt design in the setting of simultaneous 2-team approach, which is widely implemented in many centers involved in head and neck reconstruction nowadays, necessitates effective communication between the reconstructive team members and ablation team colleagues.

Reversibility of the design effective at any time is also important (discussed later).

Erroneous Execution Definition

Erroneous execution refers to a fault in recipient vessels preparation, flap harvest, flap inset, and/or microanastomosis. Because the focus of this article is not flap failure, only flap harvest with focus on reversibility is addressed, and faulty flap inset that may lead to adversity in reconstruction is focused on.

Despite thorough planning and design, reversibility should be maintained to accommodate sudden changes in the resection plan, preventing faulty flap harvest.

Using the 2 workhorse flaps in head and neck reconstruction, the ALT flap and the fibula osteoseptocutaneous flap, as examples, reversibility can be maintained throughout the harvest by leaving one side of the skin paddle uncut until the end of surgery and after checking the defect surface area and volume. This can easily be done during the ALT flap harvest, and the anterior approach for harvesting the fibula osteoseptocutaneous flap can further facilitate it.[17]

Reversibility also means the ability to add a muscle component, when needed, in particular, when it is not initially planned or designed. This is better addressed at the end of flap harvest by maintaining the integrity of the descending branch during ALT flap harvest and avoiding clipping branches to the soleus muscle during fibula flap harvest via an anterior approach.[14,18] Keeping the distal runoff of the descending branch of the lateral circumflex femoral artery also preserves other skin vessels in case a perforator injury is encountered. Other anatomic variations, which are not uncommon but not in the scope of this article, are better discussed with an experienced surgeon before proceeding with flap harvest to avoid irreversible damage.

Inset is the part of execution that demands tremendous skills and expertise. It is when all elements of the reconstruction are put into action, with a surgeon's mind connecting the present defect with its potential condition postsurgery and radiotherapy.

Inset, in authors hands, is done in a freestyle manner, instead of following a defect template. Although experience demanding, the freestyle

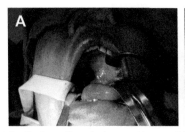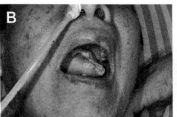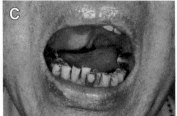

Fig. 3. Poor flap design and inset with initially poor result. Good final appearance and function after flap revision. (*A*) The defect involved 50% of the soft palate. (*B*) Unacceptable bulky flap in the palate. (*C*) Good flap appearance and speech at 2 years' follow-up after revision surgery.

manner allows individuality in the reconstruction with a subjective tendency to reconstruct structures slightly bigger compared with the approach of using a precise template; this could be helpful to counter tissue atrophy and the effect of radiotherapy. Creativity is another particular advantage of freestyle inset; many genuine ideas are born around the time the flap is ready for inset.

Case 3: good execution

A 67-year-old male patient, whose history was significant for right buccal cancer (T4aN1M0) for which he received an ALT flap in 2001, and a second primary cancer (T2N0M0) at the right buccal for which he received another ALT flap in 2015, presented with a third primary tumor at the left buccal T1N0M0 in 2016. He received buccal and mouth floor excision in addition to marginal mandibulectomy from parasymphysis to angle. The reconstruction was achieved by soft tissue flap; profunda femoris artery perforator flap, and due to previous radiotherapy and skeletonization of the mandible after marginal mandibulectomy, the risk of mandibular necrosis was high; therefore, the flap was split along the Scarpa fascia to wrap the mandible with 2-layer of vascularized tissue (**Fig. 4**).

Case 4: poor execution

A 54-year-old male patient was diagnosed in 2012 with left buccal squamous cell carcinoma, T4bN2bM0. He received composite segmental mandibulectomy from midline to subcondyle, and the reconstruction was achieved by double free flaps, a fibula osteoseptocutaneous flap for bone and oral lining reconstruction, and

ALT myocutaneous flap for skin and volume augmentation.

The ALT myocutaneous flap was not inset properly and that resulted in the flap sagging and losing most of its effective bulk, which necessitated multiple revision surgeries and secondary free flap reconstruction for augmentation (**Fig. 5**).

At the end, erroneous inset is the product of inexperience/lack of supervision or due to defective planning and inapt design. It is unfortunate that until this date there are no good resources to illustrate this part of the surgery in an easy to understand, easy to follow manner.

Highlighting the unfavorable results from around the world, however, may help surgeons to perform reconstruction better.

THE AUTHORS' MODEL TO MINIMIZE THE LIKELIHOOD OF UNFAVORABLE RECONSTRUCTION

The senior surgeon, a long time ago, established a whiteboard morning ritual, during which the team members gather in the morning of the surgery to discuss the case and finalize the surgical plan. This has evolved into an electronic patient-profile book that grants enough space to elaborate on the oncologic aspects of the case, prognosis, and ablation plan and provide detailed reconstructive plan with comparison between plan A and bailout plans. Illustrations are rich and make understanding of the surgery easier. The 10-minute presentation augments the World Health Organization regulations of patient safety, provokes a thorough discussion that often leads to innovation of an approach or

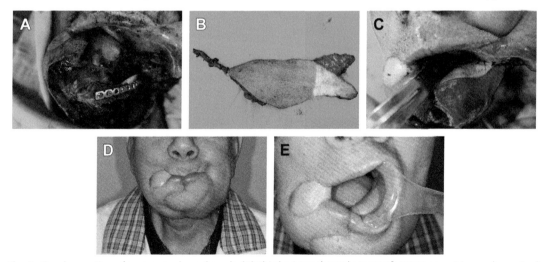

Fig. 4. Good execution of surgery and good result. (*A*) Third primary buccal cancer after tumor excision and marginal mandibulectomy. A reconstruction plate was used to reinforce the remaining thin left mandible. (*B, C*) The ALT flap was split into 2 layers along the Scarpa fascia with the skin layer de-epithelized to cover both reconstruction plate and the entire exposed marginal mandibulectomy. (*D, E*) Good appearance and function after 1-year follow-up.

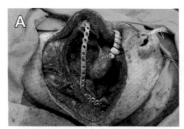
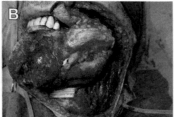
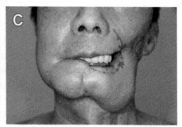
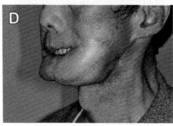

Fig. 5. Poor execution, poor initial appearance, and good final appearance after another free flap augmentation. (*A*) Composite segmental mandibulectomy with preformed plate followed by double flap reconstruction (fibula osteoseptocutaneous + ALT). (*B*) Inset of the second flap (ALT myocutanous flap). Note the muscle was nicely wrapped around the plate with the soft tissue defect in neck and maxillary area were left inadequately replaced. (*C*) Despite several revisions, the cheek remained sunken in 2014. (*D*) Good final appearance at 2 years after another free flap augmentation in 2016.

technique or provides a basis for a meaningful research, and has all the team members engaged with clear assignments. It also provides a long-lasting record of the cases for trainees to follow and learn by a constant feedback.

REFERENCES

1. Hanasono MM, Friel MT, Klem C, et al. Impact of reconstructive microsurgery in patients with advanced oral cavity cancers. Head Neck 2009; 31(10):1289–96.

2. Lin CS, Jen YM, Kao WY, et al. Improved outcomes in buccal squamous cell carcinoma. Head Neck 2013;35(1):65–71.

3. Amit M, Yen TC, Liao CT, et al, International Consortium for Outcome Research (ICOR) in Head and Neck Cancer. Improvement in survival of patients with oral cavity squamous cell carcinoma: an international collaborative study. Cancer 2013;119(24):4242–8.

4. Hanasono MM, Corbitt CA, Yu P, et al. Success of sequential free flaps in head and neck reconstruction. J Plast Reconstr Aesthet Surg 2014;67(9):1186–93.

5. Zaghi S, Danesh J, Hendizadeh L, et al. Changing indications for maxillomandibular reconstruction with osseous free flaps: a 17-year experience with 620 consecutive cases at UCLA and the impact of osteoradionecrosis. Laryngoscope 2014;124(6):1329–35.

6. Markey J, Knott PD, Fritz MA, et al. Recent advances in head and neck free tissue transfer. Curr Opin Otolaryngol Head Neck Surg 2015; 23(4):297–301.

7. Pierre CS, Dassonville O, Chamorey E, et al. Long-term functional outcomes and quality of life after oncologic surgery and microvascular reconstruction in patients with oral or oropharyngeal cancer. Acta Otolaryngol 2014;134(10):1086–93.

8. Fujioka M, Masuda K, Imamura Y. Fatty tissue atrophy of free flap used for head and neck reconstruction. Microsurgery 2011;31(1):32–5.

9. Lambade PN, Lambade D, Goel M. Osteoradionecrosis of the mandible: a review. Oral Maxillofac Surg 2013;17(4):243–9.

10. Wallace CG, Chang YM, Tsai CY, et al. Harnessing the potential of the free fibula osteoseptocutaneous flap in mandible reconstruction. Plast Reconstr Surg 2010;125(1):305–14.

11. Wong CH, Wei FC. Microsurgical free flap in head and neck reconstruction. Head Neck 2010;32(9): 1236–45.

12. Wei FC, Jain V, Celik N, et al. Have we found an ideal soft-tissue flap? an experience with 672 anterolateral thigh flaps. Plast Reconstr Surg 2002;109(7): 2219–26 [discussion: 2227–30].

13. Wei FC, Seah CS, Tsai YC, et al. Fibula osteoseptocutaneous flap for reconstruction of composite mandibular defects. Plast Reconstr Surg 1994; 93(2):294–304 [discussion: 305–6].

14. Ali RS, Bluebond-Langner R, Rodriguez ED, et al. The versatility of the anterolateral thigh flap. Plast Reconstr Surg 2009;124(6 Suppl):e395–407.

15. Hallock GG. Simplified nomenclature for compound flaps. Plast Reconstr Surg 2000;105(4):1465–70 [quiz: 1471–2].

16. Hallock GG. The complete nomenclature for combined perforator flaps. Plast Reconstr Surg 2011; 127(4):1720–9.

17. Wei FC, Chen HC, Chuang CC, et al. Fibular osteoseptocutaneous flap:anatomic study and clinical application. Plast Reconstr Surg 1986;78(2):191–200.

18. Cheng MH, Saint-Cyr M, Ali RS, et al. Osteomyocutaneous peroneal artery-based combined flap for reconstruction of composite and en bloc mandibular defects. Head Neck 2009;31(3):361–70.

Free Tissue Transfer to Head and Neck

Lessons Learned from Unfavorable Results—Experience per Subsite

Nidal Farhan AL Deek, MSc, MD, Fu-Chan Wei, MD*, Huang-Kai Kao, MD

KEYWORDS

- Free tissue transfer • Microsurgical head and neck recosntruction • Unfavorable results
- Complications

KEY POINTS

- Unfavorable microsurgical head and neck reconstruction refers to complicated wound healing and suboptimal form and function despite free flap survival.
- The unique characteristics of some of the anatomic subsites and the unavailability of optimal techniques contribute to the unfavorable result.
- Knowing when to offer a priority reconstruction and when to do total reconstruction per site can reduce unfavorable outcomes.
- The reconstructive surgeon should foresee the effect of surgical scar contracture, radiotherapy, and the extent of tissue atrophy on the reconstruction and take necessary countermeasures.

INTRODUCTION

Free tissue transfer after ablation of head and neck cancer has become the gold standard of reconstruction.[1] In order for the microsurgical reconstruction to achieve its ultimate goal of good patient quality of life, successfully transferred free flaps should aim at restoring optimal form and function.

Good quality of life after head and neck reconstruction depends on uncomplicated wound healing to allow timely administration of chemotherapy and radiotherapy; adequate mouth opening, good deglutition, and intelligible speech; minimal donor site morbidity; minimal revision surgeries; and good cosmesis.[2,3] Fulfilling these goals demands thorough planning, wise and proper selection of techniques, and flawless execution of the surgery to ensure successful reconstruction beyond free flap survival.

Failure in achieving one or more of these goals despite successful free flap transfer results in unfavorable reconstruction marked with downgraded quality of life. Avoidance and treatment of the unfavorable results thus should be at the core of contemporary head and neck surgery.

The authors of this article, based on their extensive experience, identify potential challenges and pitfalls by region or anatomic structure in the head and neck and share their refined approach in a lesson-learned manner.

The authors have no conflict of interest to declare.

Department of Plastic and Reconstructive Surgery, Chang Gung Memorial Hospital, Chang Gung Medical College, Chang Gung University, 199 Tun-Hwa North Road, Taipei 10591, Taiwan

* Corresponding author.

E-mail address: fuchanwei@gmail.com

Clin Plastic Surg 43 (2016) 621–630
http://dx.doi.org/10.1016/j.cps.2016.06.003
0094-1298/16/$ – see front matter © 2016 Elsevier Inc. All rights reserved.

UNFAVORABLE RESULTS AFTER MICROSURGICAL RECONSTRUCTION OF TONGUE AND MOUTH FLOOR DEFECTS
Unfavorable Results

Untoward outcomes after microsurgical reconstruction of the tongue and mouth floor involve inadequate volume reconstruction of the neotongue; strictures and tethering of the tongue; orocutaneous fistula; and/or suboptimal management of associating bony and/or soft tissue defect involving the mandible, palate, and lateral pharyngeal wall.[4]

Radiotherapy negatively affects the reconstruction, and the effect of radiotherapy on the flap and surrounding tissue is unpredictable and hard to control. Therefore, it seems logical to foresee the aftermath of radiotherapy to minimize related shortcomings and complications.

Classification of Tongue Defects

To avoid confusion, the authors refer to 50% loss of the tongue in anterior-to-posterior direction as hemiglossectomy and to more than 90% loss of the tongue with preservation of less than 10% of tongue base as near-total glossectomy. Total tongue defect refers to total resection of the tongue with/without the hyoid bone.

Other forms of tongue defects or defects not limited to the tongue, extending to mouth floor and adjacent structures, represent a largely diverse group that lacks uniformity and is better addressed individually.

Revisited Approach

On hemiglossectomy
Tethering-free reconstruction and water-tight closure at mouth floor are the goals.[5] The authors prefer thin anterolateral thigh cutaneous flap[6] to ensure pliable, soft neohemitongue. The flap is harvested above the deep fascia or the scarpa fascia depending on patient's thigh thickness.[7,8] During inset, the flap is sutured from posterior to anterior starting with the lateral side of the lower gum, then the tongue side leaving the anterior ventral tongue and anterior side of the lower gum toward the end. This allows the redundant part of the flap to be de-epithelialized to augment the neotongue with tension-free closure. Before closure and with care not to injure skin vessels, the inner side of the flap is sutured to the intrinsic muscles of the tongue to separate between mouth floor and oral tongue creating oral gutter (**Fig. 1**).

On near-total and total glossectomies
The key goals are to achieve long-lasting bulky neotongue with protective sensation, allow

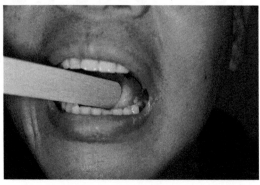

Fig. 1. Adequate gutter between tongue and lower gum after reconstruction of hemiglossectomy defect with thin anterolateral thigh flap.

decanulation of the tracheostomy, and reasonable swallowing. The flap of choice is the combined anterolateral thigh flap with vastus lateralis muscle. Any flap with similar characteristics and tissue component can also be used.

The anterolateral thigh flap allows stocky neotongue given that the flap is not stretched too thin to reconstruct every soft tissue defect in the oral cavity, such as the palatine tonsillar fossa or the soft palate. The vastus lateralis muscle is designed along the distal runoff of the descending branch to allow versatile obliteration of the dead space between the mandible and the hyoid bone.

Flap inset starts with the epiglottis all the way up along the lateral pharyngeal wall, then the flap is folded on itself anteriorly to create bulky tongue and finally sutured to the mandible/plate to seal the mouth floor. The next important step is hyoid bone suspension to the mandible/reconstruction plate, which opens up the epiglottis and lifts up the hyoid bone and the bottom of the flap minimizing sagging and flap sinking caused by gravity and bottoming out. The lateral cutaneous femoral nerve is coapted to the lingual nerve to provide protective sensation.

The presence of associating segmental mandibulectomy further complicates the reconstruction.[9] The authors recommend another free flap to address these defects.[10] This is discussed further in the section on mandible reconstruction (**Fig. 2**).

UNFAVORABLE RESULTS AFTER MICROSURGICAL RECONSTRUCTION OF THE MANDIBLE
Unfavorable Results

The untoward outcomes are soft tissue–related and bone- and hardware-related. In the first category, sunken appearance and orocutaneous fistula are

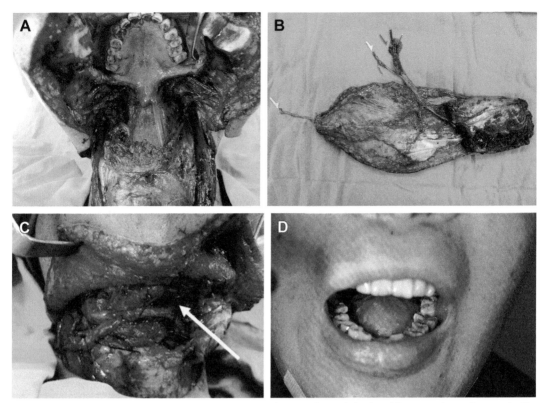

Fig. 2. (*A*) Total glossectomy defect. (*B*) The combined anterolateral thigh with vastus lateralis muscle flap including the motor nerve and the sensory nerve. (*C*) Inset of the flap for total tongue reconstruction with hyoid bone suspension (*arrow*). (*D*) Appearance after reconstruction with good shape and function at 1-year follow-up.

the main unfavorable results.[11,12] In the second category, malocclusion, plate exposure, trismus, and asymmetric appearance are the main problems.[11,12]

The untoward outcomes following the reconstruction of the mandible arise largely from poor decision making; in particular, whether or not to reconstruct the bone and failing to appreciate the importance of adequate volume replacement and soft tissue coverage. Other aspects of poor decision making include whether or not to plate and failure to prioritize reconstruction goals in the setting of an extensive defect, building on a deceiving concept: "One flap can do many things."

Revisited Approach

To avoid poor decision making leading to inadequate or overzealous reconstruction, a refined multifactorial approach, that of the patient, the disease, and the defect elements, has been adopted into our practice. Based on this approach, the suitable reconstructive plan consists of vascularized bone alone, soft tissue flap with or without reconstruction plate, and double free flap (vascularized bone plus soft tissue flap). The reconstruction is done in either one-stage when a full-scope reconstructive effort is desired based on favorable general and oncologic conditions, proper defect type, and good mouth opening; or in multistage starting with soft tissue first, then bone reconstruction later when a full-scope endeavor is deemed unsuitable, in contract to that of one-stage reconstruction (**Fig. 3**).

Special Considerations

Defect classification

Defect type based on Jewer's[13] and Wei's classification[14,15] does not necessarily preclude the bony reconstruction; instead, these classifications are used as a guideline for potential compromise in the reconstruction plan when other factors, such as prognosis and mouth opening, are unfavorable; for example, an L compound defect in poor prognosis tumors may be best reconstructed with soft tissue flap with or without plate depending on the severity of trismus. However, the same defect following ameloblastoma resection is best reconstructed with vascularized bone.

The reconstruction plate

Although the reconstruction plate maintains the continuity of the mandible, it could be a double-edge

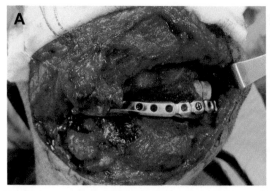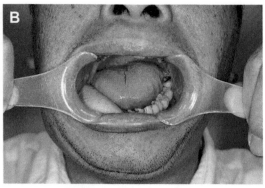

Fig. 3. One-stage reconstruction of a compound mandibular defect. (*A*) The compound mandibular defect after excision of ameloblastoma with preformed reconstruction plate. (*B*) Appearance at 1-year follow-up after one-stage reconstruction with the fibula osteoseptocutaneous free flap.

sword leading to complications; exposure is not uncommon, not to mention malocclusion, trismus, and asymmetry. To minimize plate-related complications, the authors advocate plate-free reconstruction in the case of long-standing severe trismus with a history of radiotherapy or osteoradionecrosis, because the mandible is less likely to drift after resection and plate-free reconstruction.

The recently available preformed plate (Matrix-Mandible, Synthes CMF, West Chester, PA) allows anatomic and symmetric restoration of the shape of the mandible with ease and minimal or no bending. The plate is suitable for a wide array of mandibular defects except central (C type) and bilateral defects (LCL type).

High osteotomies and condyle head

The main concern following high mandibulectomy is condyle head malposition after fixation. Malpositioned condyle head leads to locked jaw and pain. To avoid that, intraoperative navigation to register the location of the condyle head before resection and then to use the registered location as a landmark for plate fixation can be used, or a miniplate can be fixed to the condyle head and to the zygoma/maxilla before segmental resection, so that when plating is done, the condyle is already in the anatomic location (**Fig. 4**). When none of these techniques is feasible, the condyle head could be pushed upward and backward to ensure its proper position in the glenoid fossa.

UNFAVORABLE RESULTS AFTER MICROSURGICAL RECONSTRUCTION OF THE MAXILLA
Unfavorable Results

The untoward outcomes following the microsurgical reconstruction of a maxillary defect are largely oronasal or oronasocutaneous fistula.

Diplopia is another possible complication when the orbital floor is involved in resection without adequate support at the time of reconstruction. To a lesser degree, the loss of midfacial height and projection can also be considered among unfavorable results from a cosmetic point of view.[16,17]

Revisited Approach

The question "to reconstruct the bone or not" is the key question that affects flap selection and subsequent outcomes. Most of the reported unfavorable outcomes are the result of faulty answers.

Because the maxillary defect is generally variable involving multiple anatomic structures[16] that are difficult to reconstruct at once, especially with single flap,[16] it should be a top priority approach to the reconstruction instead of an attempt to reconstruct everything.[18]

Although there are several classifications of maxillary defects, and some of them are comprehensive covering all defect scenarios, none of

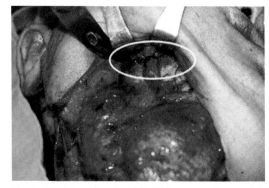

Fig. 4. Miniplate fixation (*circle*) between the condyle head and the maxilla before segmental resection was done to avoid malposition.

them is a clear approach. Therefore we propose a top-priority-oriented approach as follows. When the top-priority goals are total dead space obliteration, water-tight separation between skull base and sinonasal cavities, and long-lasting orbital support, they are preferably achieved by a soft tissue flap and orbital mesh leaving buttress reconstruction for a secondary stage. The involvement of the external skin or the extent of the defect to the contralateral maxilla further increases the soft tissue and volume loss justifying a soft tissue flap.

At a secondary stage, the buttress in need for reconstruction is identified and a bony flap is provided. This approach avoids unfavorable results including fistula and trismus because it is difficult trying to address all the variables (bone and soft tissue) within the limited space of the maxilla. This approach represents a signature lesson-learned approach, because complications usually arise from soft tissue and coverage (**Fig. 5**).

When the top-priority goal is not dead space obliteration, volume replacement, and separation of spaces/cavities, but rather facial projection

and height and dental restoration based on the extent of the maxillary alveolar arch involvement with attention to the canine,[16] then osteoseptocutaneous fibula flap reconstruction is preferred.

Special Considerations

Orbital support is achieved by different means; however, the authors prefer orbital mesh because it does not suffer from resorption, does not result in increased rate of infection, and is easy to contour.[19] A three-dimensional print of the contralateral orbit may further increase the speed and precision in mesh contouring.[20]

When orbital support and dead space obliteration are important, it is vital to foresee the inevitable tissue atrophy and possible sagging of the flap. Therefore, the authors prefer fasciocutaneous over myocutaneous flap, because the latter has more significant volume loss resulting in hardware exposure, fistula, or even diplopia. When the anterolateral thigh skin flap is used for this purpose, even it is thin, the flap still can be

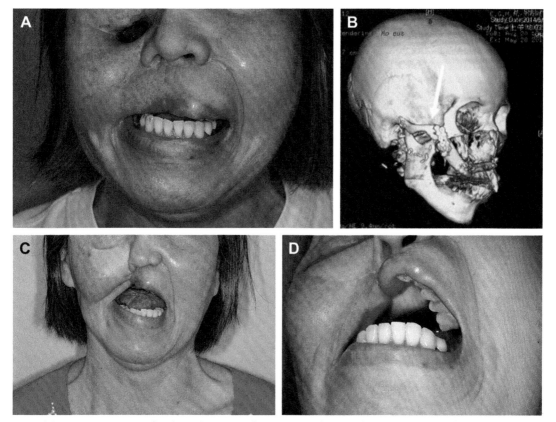

Fig. 5. (*A*) Oronasocutaneous fistula with trismus after excision of adenoid cystic carcinoma of the maxillary sinus with immediate fibula flap reconstruction. (*B*) Three-dimensional computed tomography shows the fibula strut impinged on the coronoid process locking the lower jaw (*arrow*). (*C, D*) Result after burring down the interfering fibula strut and coronoidotomy along with fistula obliteration and external face reconstruction with anterolateral thigh flap at 1-year follow-up.

de-epithelialized and stacked to obliterate the dead space and isolate and seal cavities or spaces. The fascia can be used as a sling to further suspend the tissues and prevent sagging.

UNFAVORABLE RESULTS AFTER MICROSURGICAL RECONSTRUCTION OF THE ORAL LINING, SOFT PALATE, LIPS, AND ORAL COMMISSURE
Oral Lining

Unfavorable results
The oral lining is understated in microsurgical head and neck reconstruction despite the key role it plays in mouth opening, saliva secretion, and the oropharyngeal substitute's function.[21] Therefore, untoward outcomes are diverse including xerostomia; trismus; reduced oral cavity volume; and tethering of the dynamic structures, such as the lips, tongue, and soft palate with compromised function leading to drooling, nasal regurgitation, nasality, dysphagia, and so forth.

The unique characteristics of the oral mucosa
The mucosal lining presents a formidable challenge in itself that is responsible to some extent, given its unique and diverse nature, for the suboptimal result after reconstruction. For example, the oral lining is heterogeneous. Different histologic characteristics between secretory and nonsecretory and mobile and nonmobile mucosa exist, which affect the role the mucosa lining play per site. Moreover, the postablative defect usually spans multiple oral mucosa subsites of different form and function, such as the tongue and mouth floor, the buccal and mouth floor, the lip, the buccal and the palate, or any similar combination. Therefore, "like-with like" reconstruction could be complex, if not impossible.

Revisited approach
Our experience with oral mucosa resurfacing includes skin flaps that are pliable, thin, and sensate but not secretory; muscle flaps that develop rapid mucosalization and have good appearance, but are neither sensate nor lubricative; and colonic mucosa that can produce mucins for lubrication, but are too sticky, prone to hypertrophy, and their donor site morbidity is far from being negligible.

An optimal method to reconstruct the oral mucosa may not be available yet; therefore, the following notes should be considered when selecting the reconstructive technique. Whenever possible, and to minimize tethering, oral mucosa subsites should not always be addressed with one flap; for example, nondependent areas that play no dynamic role could be left to heal by secondary intention, if tethering may occur with one-flap reconstruction.

Furthermore, muscle flaps are more prone to fibrosis and they are not suitable for the reconstruction of mobile and pliable mucosa, such as the buccal mucosa or the soft palate (**Fig. 6**). Skin flaps without inclusion of underneath fascia are good for these defects, because the fascia may become fibrotic and stiff resulting in limitation of mouth opening. Regardless of the flap used for resurfacing, the flap cannot be too bulky to avoid autochewing, which may induce inflammation and scaring that eventually leads to trismus. The colonic flaps are out of our favor because of the previously shortcomings, but they are still indicated in circular esophageal defects and voice reconstruction.

The Palate

The unfavorable results
Reconstruction of the palate may affect quality of speech and contribute to or prevent nasal

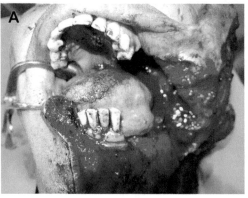
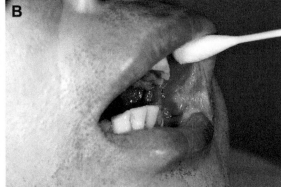

Fig. 6. (*A*) The oral mucosa defect after cancer excision involved inferior maxilla, trigone, and buccal mucosa. (*B*) Trismus and muscle hypertrophy after reconstruction with vastus lateralis muscle only and spontaneous mucosalization over the muscle.

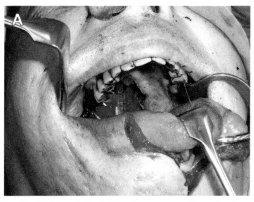 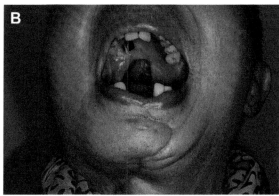

Fig. 7. (A) The defect after tumor resection also involved soft and hard palate and inferior maxilla. (B) Oronasal fistula and oropharyngeal deficiency after radial forearm flap reconstruction.

regurgitation.[21] The complex musculatures found in the dynamic anatomic structure, particularly in the soft palate, are too difficult to be addressed with one flap whether cutaneous, muscular, or musculocutaneous,[2] not to mention that the extent of resection decreases postoperative outcomes.[22,23] The weight of the flap and gravity effect may easily cause dehiscence between the flap and the native tissue resulting in oronasal fistula (**Fig. 7**).

Revisited approach
Soft palate We divide a soft palatal defect into subtotal (<75%), near total, and total (>75%).

For subtotal defects, the soft palate remnant is stretched as much as possible and sutured to the lateral pharyngeal wall only from the posterior side to narrow the velopharynx. The anterior side, which is now continuous, is resurfaced with thin cutaneous flap only.[22] For more than 75% or total soft palate defects, a thin fasciocutaneous flap is used. The skin is used for oral lining, and the fascia is for nasal lining. The flap can be folded on itself partially only when the pedicle needs to be protected from the nasal airway to avoid desiccation or infection. Meticulous repair with the mucosa of the hard palate is important to avoid dehiscence at the suture line and fistula (**Fig. 8**).

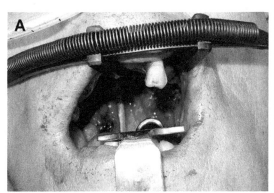 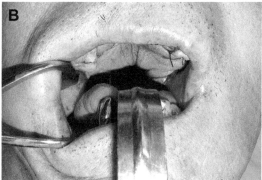

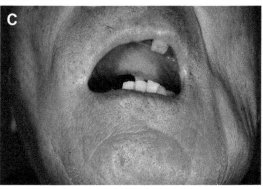

Fig. 8. (A) The defect after tumor resection involved total soft palate. (B) Flap inset, the flap was partly folded to protect the pedicle from being exposed to airway. (C) At 1-year follow-up.

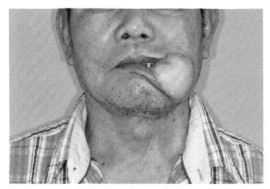

Fig. 9. Downward malpositioned lower lip with notable oral incompetency.

To improve the velopharyngeal function, a pharyngeal flap, superiorly or inferiorly based, at later stage after completion of radiotherapy is used.

Hard palate Although skin flaps can reconstruct the defect, they largely result in patchy appearance; therefore, we have grown more in favor of muscle flap reconstruction with care to prevent flap sagging in the oral cavity and subsequent dehiscence and oronasal fistula.

Lip and Oral Commissure

Unfavorable results

The untoward outcomes involve oral incompetency and drooling, downward malpositioned lower lip, upward malpositioned upper lip, microstomia, and shallow or absent lip-alveolar sulcus (**Fig. 9**).

Revisited approach

To avoid untoward outcomes, the issues that need to be addressed may include the extent of lower lip resection and the need for postoperative radiotherapy. When the lower lip is largely intact, using a tougher flap and anchoring the remaining lip high on the flap helps counter pull-down effect from the flap weight and gravity. No suspension is required. However, when the lower lip has significantly lost its height and width, suspension of the flap to prevent a down-positioned lip-flap complex postoperatively may become necessary (**Fig. 10**).

In through-and-through cheek defects involving oral commissure, we prefer to fold the flap on itself to create a bulky commissure, which facilitates secondary revision, especially when postoperative radiotherapy is needed (**Fig. 11**). Unless the defect is shallow, not including substantial loss of the orbicularis oris, or there is a need to recreate the

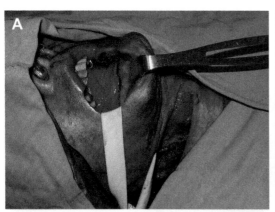

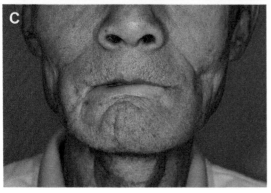

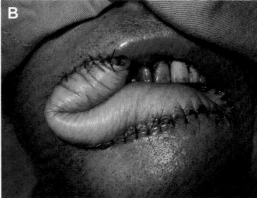

Fig. 10. (*A*) The defect after tumor resection. (*B*) Flap inset. (*C*) Good appearance and oral competency at 5-year follow-up.

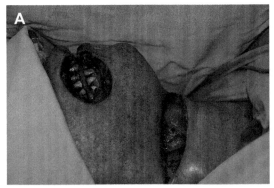

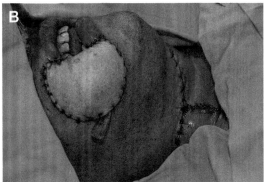

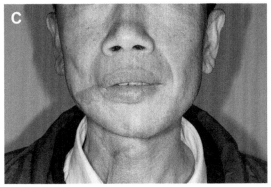

Fig. 11. (*A*) The defect involved the oral commissure, upper and lower lip, and through-and-through cheek. (*B*) Flap inset and appearance at the end of reconstruction. (*C*) Good cosmesis and oral competency after flap revision at 2-year follow-up.

labiogingival sulcus, the radial forearm flap has fallen out of our favor because the tissue rigidity of the radial forearm is not as strong as the anterolateral thigh flap.

When radiotherapy is indicated, the authors prefer not to optimize lip and commissure reconstruction initially because of the unpredictable contracture after irradiation. Tendon- or fascial-based sling reconstruction is better avoided because after contracture of the tendon/fascial sling occurs, it becomes hard to correct.

SUMMARY

Good quality of life depends on uncomplicated wound healing and optimal restoration of form and function. Unfavorable results downgrade a patient's quality of life and should be avoided by optimization of the surgical plan, design, and execution. They are as important as achieving disease-free survival and successful free tissue transfer at this advanced stage of free flap surgery.

Although one-stage total reconstruction is trendy and desirable, extensive and complex head and neck defects may need to be approached in a staged manner, taking into account all the priorities. Keeping reconstruction priorities clear and avoiding multipurpose shooting with single flap in one stage helps minimize the unfavorable outcomes.

Bulk restoration remains the ultimate goal in tongue reconstruction, but maintaining the bulk is the challenge until now. For oral lining, there is no optimal technique; unfavorable outcomes are inevitable. However, every effort should be taken to minimize complications resulting from selected techniques. In mandibular and maxillary defects, whether or not to reconstruct the bone and to do one- or two-stage reconstruction are the key questions. Although clinicians strive to achieve one-stage total reconstruction, it is best to remain realistic because this goal may not be achievable. Therefore, a multifactorial consideration that addresses the prognosis, the extent of surgery, and the patient's functional needs and cosmesis may influence the final decision.

REFERENCES

1. Sakuraba M, Miyamoto S, Kimata Y, et al. Recent advances in reconstructive surgery: head and neck reconstruction. Int J Clin Oncol 2013;18(4): 561–5.
2. Markey J, Knott PD, Fritz MA, et al. Recent advances in head and neck free tissue transfer. Curr Opin Otolaryngol Head Neck Surg 2015;23(4): 297–301.

3. Pierre CS, Dassonville O, Chamorey E, et al. Long-term functional outcomes and quality of life after oncologic surgery and microvascular reconstruction in patients with oral or oropharyngeal cancer. Acta Otolaryngol 2014;134(10):1086–93.

4. Chang EI, Yu P, Skoracki RJ, et al. Comprehensive analysis of functional outcomes and survival after microvascular reconstruction of glossectomy defects. Ann Surg Oncol 2015;22(9):3061–9.

5. Engel H, Huang JJ, Lin CY, et al. A strategic approach for tongue reconstruction to achieve predictable and improved functional and aesthetic outcomes. Plast Reconstr Surg 2010;126(6):1967–77.

6. Wong CH, Wei FC. Anterolateral thigh flap. Head Neck 2010;32(4):529–40.

7. Wei FC, Jain V, Celik N, et al. Have we found an ideal soft-tissue flap? An experience with 672 anterolateral thigh flaps. Plast Reconstr Surg 2002;109(7): 2219–26 [discussion: 2227–30].

8. Hong JP, Chung IW. The superficial fascia as a new plane of elevation for anterolateral thigh flaps. Ann Plast Surg 2013;70(2):192–5.

9. Hanasono MM, Weinstock YE, Yu P. Reconstruction of extensive head and neck defects with multiple simultaneous free flaps. Plast Reconstr Surg 2008; 122(6):1739–46.

10. Wallace CG, Tsao CK, Wei FC. Role of multiple free flaps in head and neck reconstruction. Curr Opin Otolaryngol Head Neck Surg 2014;22(2):140–6.

11. Hidalgo DA, Pusic AL. Free-flap mandibular reconstruction: a 10-year follow-up study. Plast Reconstr Surg 2002;110(2):438–49 [discussion: 450–1].

12. Pirgousis P, Eberle N, Fernandes R. Reoperative mandibular reconstruction. Oral Maxillofac Surg Clin North Am 2011;23(1):153–60, vii.

13. Jewer DD, Boyd JB, Manktelow RT, et al. Orofacial and mandibular reconstruction with the iliac crest free flap: a review of 60 cases and a new method of classification. Plast Reconstr Surg 1989;84(3): 391–403 [discussion: 404–5].

14. Wei FC, Demirkan F, Chen HC, et al. Double free flaps in reconstruction of extensive composite mandibular defects in head and neck cancer. Plast Reconstr Surg 1999;103(1):39–47.

15. Probst FA, Mast G, Ermer M, et al. MatrixMANDIBLE preformed reconstruction plates–a two-year two-institution experience in 71 patients. J Oral Maxillofac Surg 2012;70(11):e657–66.

16. Hanasono MM, Silva AK, Yu P, et al. A comprehensive algorithm for oncologic maxillary reconstruction. Plast Reconstr Surg 2013;131(1): 47–60.

17. Cordeiro PG, Chen CM. A 15-year review of midface reconstruction after total and subtotal maxillectomy: part I. Algorithm and outcomes. Plast Reconstr Surg 2012;129(1):124–36.

18. Archibald S, Jackson S, Thoma A. Paranasal sinus and midfacial reconstruction. Clin Plast Surg 2005; 32:309–25.

19. Kirby EJ, Turner JB, Davenport DL, et al. Orbital floor fractures: outcomes of reconstruction. Ann Plast Surg 2011;66:508–12.

20. Mustafa SF, Evans PL, Bocca A, et al. Customized titanium reconstruction of post-traumatic orbital wall defects: a review of 22 cases. Int J Oral Maxillofac Surg 2011;40(12):1357–62.

21. Rigby MH, Taylor SM. Soft tissue reconstruction of the oral cavity: a review of current options. Curr Opin Otolaryngol Head Neck Surg 2013;21(4): 311–7.

22. Moerman M, Vermeersch H, Van Lierde K, et al. Refinement of the free radial forearm flap reconstructive technique after resection of large oropharyngeal malignancies with excellent functional results. Head Neck 2003;25(9):772–7.

23. Jeng SF, Kuo YR, Wei FC, et al. Reconstruction of concomitant lip and cheek through-and-through defects with combined free flap and an advancement flap from the remaining lip. Plast Reconstr Surg 2004;113(2):491–8.

Mount Sinai Medical Center and Their Experience with Unfavorable Microsurgical Head and Neck Reconstruction

Ilya Likhterov, MD[a],*, Mark Urken, MD[b]

KEYWORDS

• Salvage • Postradiation • Laryngopharyngeal reconstruction • Salivary leak • Complications

KEY POINTS

- Reconstruction of the head and neck defects in a salvage setting increases the risks of complications.
- Protection of the vascular pedicle from a potential salivary leak is paramount to success of the reconstructive effort.
- Elimination of dead space and selection of suitable donor blood vessels for the anastomosis is important.

Since the introduction of microvascular techniques in head and neck reconstruction, the field has progressed tremendously with free flap survival rates ranging from 90% to 98%.[1–3] Many factors contribute to this degree of progress. Experience of the surgeons, improved understanding of the physiologic changes associated with ischemic injury and reperfusion, preoperative patient selection, and vigilant postoperative care are essential to safely accomplish the goal of a successful reconstruction.

However, the challenges to microvascular reconstruction have increased significantly as primary radiation for head and neck malignancy has become more widely used. Salvage operations after failure of primary radiation or of multimodality treatment are common indications for free flap reconstruction. Bone containing free tissue transfer is the most reliable strategy in treatment of Grade III osteoradionecrosis (ORN).[4,5] The changing trends in the indications for free flap reconstruction were highlighted in the review of the University of California Los Angeles experience. The proportion of ORN cases increased from 1.3% of all patients undergoing maxillomandibular reconstruction from 1995 to 2000 to 8.7% from 2001 to 2006 to 17.5% from 2007 to 2012 (P<.05).[6] Thus, a surgeon who may expect a favorable outcome in a reconstruction performed in the primary setting must be prepared for, and anticipate, the obstacles that arise in the reconstruction of an ablative defect in an irradiated field performed in the salvage setting.

Here we review the lessons learned, and the key considerations for optimizing results when performing reconstruction in a patient with a previous history of head and neck radiation.

[a] Head and Neck Oncologic and Reconstructive Surgery, Department of Otolaryngology, Mount Sinai Beth Israel, 10 Union Square East, Suite 5B, New York, NY 10003, USA; [b] Division of Head and Neck Surgical Oncology, Department of Otolaryngology, Mount Sinai Beth Israel, 10 Union Square East, Suite 5B, New York, NY 10003, USA
* Corresponding author.
E-mail address: ilikhterov@chpnet.org

Clin Plastic Surg 43 (2016) 631–638
http://dx.doi.org/10.1016/j.cps.2016.05.004

RADIATION EFFECTS

Radiation effects on the tissue are well known to most clinicians treating patients with head and neck malignancies. Although early radiation-induced skin and mucosal reactions acutely affect patients during and immediately after radiation treatment, it is the delayed radiation injury that will affect long-term healing. These changes develop 4 to 6 months after completion of therapy. Epidermal atrophy and vascular and connective tissue changes leading to the loss of elasticity and fibrosis significantly reduce the pliability of soft tissues. With denser collagen fibrils and irregular elastic fibers, the tissue planes of the neck are often scarred. Lymphatic drainage is compromised with increases in postoperative edema.[7] Vascularity is impaired with thrombosis and obliteration of capillaries, resulting in poor tissue perfusion and oxygenation. Arterioles and small arteries demonstrate progressive vascular sclerosis and narrowing.[8] Periosteal blood supply to bone is compromised, placing the mandible at risk for ORN. Not only is wound healing impaired, but there is also a reduced capacity for local immunologic response, which increases the risk of infection and wound complications.[9]

SURGICAL SALVAGE

Despite the progress in the oncologic management of head and neck malignancy, rates of persistent or recurrent disease of 40% to 50% have been cited in the literature for patients with advanced-stage tumors.[10–13] Salvage surgery is, by definition, the last resort at clearing local and regional disease. Although 20% to 30% of patients with local and regional failure are candidates for surgical salvage, achieving cure remains difficult. Detection of tumor margin in an irradiated field is challenging on preoperative imaging, intraoperative inspection, and on histopathologic analysis.[14] In an irradiated field, fascial barriers are less likely to stop aggressive recurrent tumor spread, and a wider resection often must be performed than in a primary setting. As an example, after radiation exposure, the periosteum of the mandible provides less resistance to tumor invasion of the bone. Rather than infiltration through an occlusal surface alone, in an irradiated specimen, invasion is seen at multiple sites along the cortex.[15] The reduced structural support of the irradiated bone, and the higher likelihood of cortex invasion from the adjacent mucosal sites often renders marginal mandibulectomy an unfavorable option in a salvage setting. For these patients, composite resection with a resultant segmental defect is the

preferred option.[16] Similarly, recurrence or persistence in the neck may present with extensive extracapsular extension requiring sternocleidomastoid sacrifice with potential carotid artery and jugular vein exposure. The reconstructive team should anticipate and be prepared to address these extensive defects.

A systematic review of the literature suggests that there are similar rates of complications and free flap survival regardless of whether the patient had preoperative radiation therapy.[17–20] Achieving a similar degree of success in the salvage and the primary settings requires careful planning and anticipation of potential complications.

The authors follow a number of guiding principles to help avoid negative outcomes in this patient population. Here we cover considerations at the time of reconstruction, vessel and flap selection, elimination of dead space, management of wound complications, define what should be designated as a safe wound, and discuss anticipatory strategies for managing flap failure. To achieve success, it is imperative that the surgical team plan every aspect of the surgical procedure and include the potential options for surgical salvage in the event of a complication.

TIMING OF RECONSTRUCTION

When it comes to salvage of persistent or recurrent malignancy, the aggressive tumor biology dictates the scheduling of the extirpative procedure. On the other hand, the reconstructive effort may be delayed for a variety of reasons. Negative margins must be ensured, especially when adjuvant therapy options have been exhausted. The surgeon may elect to wait for the final pathology evaluation and stage the reconstruction until a later date. The benefits of this approach versus the morbidity of a separate anesthetic and temporarily open defect must be discussed in detail with the patient. In cases in which there is a high probability of recurrence, and in which visual surveillance becomes limited by the reconstruction, the delay may be extended for a considerable period of time. This approach has been advocated by some investigators for malignancies in the palato-maxillary region.[21]

Active infection has a high potential for compromising the microvascular reconstruction. This adverse environment can be seen in cases of osteomyelitis, a pathologic fracture resulting from advanced ORN of the mandible, or revision of previously failed reconstruction in which necrotic tissue must first be debrided. In these types of situations, delayed free tissue transfer, treating the patient with antibiotics, and local wound care may optimize the recipient site for successful free tissue transfer as a staged procedure.

More often than not, however, the reconstruction has to be performed without delay to avoid extensive morbidity, additional scarring, and to optimize the functional outcome with the most rapid restoration of the quality of life.

VESSEL SELECTION

Exposure to radiation can induce arteritis and fibrosis of the surrounding tissue bed. Radiation for malignancies of the oral cavity and oropharynx can result in significant damage to the branches of the external carotid artery. In addition, blood vessels may be absent as a result of prior neck dissection, leaving the reconstructive surgeon with limited options in a vessel-depleted neck. As mentioned previously, the key to success in a salvage effort is anticipation of potential complications. A leak resulting from poor healing of the intraoral suture lines places any anastomosis located in the upper neck at risk. Exposure to saliva and infection can be minimized by placing the anastomosis in a more remote location, away from a potential drainage pathway from the oral cavity. This can be successfully accomplished by using the transverse cervical artery (TCA). Not only is this vessel outside of the radiation field in most patients, it can also be found in a previously undissected region of the lower neck. Distal dissection, deep to the trapezius muscle, followed by transposition of the TCA can provide favorable vessel geometry with a vertical orientation of the pedicle in the neck. In elderly patients, the TCA is less prone to significant atherosclerotic disease.[22] Another novel option for the arterial supply to the flap in a vessel-depleted neck is the internal mammary artery.[23] The inferior thyroid artery also should be considered as a potential candidate.

Recipient veins for flap drainage also may prove to be scarce in the cervical region in a salvage, postradiation setting. The transverse cervical vein can be used along with the TCA, although it is often of small caliber. Internal mammary veins become a good option when the artery is harvested in the intercostal space (**Fig. 1**).[24] In addition, the cephalic vein can be followed in the deltopectoral groove toward the upper arm and transposed into the neck.[25] This maneuver brings a good caliber vein into the neck, avoiding the need for a vein graft. Vessel selection is done on a case-by-case basis, and the surgeon should be prepared to use the options listed previously, extend the anastomosis to the contralateral neck, and use arterial and venous grafts when appropriate. The key to avoiding complications at this step of the reconstruction is to optimize the recipient artery

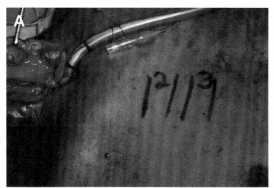

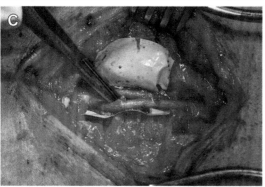

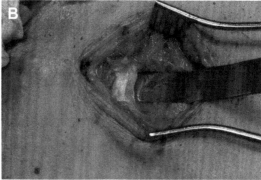

Fig. 1. (*A*) Second and third ribs are marked in preparation for the harvest of the internal mammary vessels in a patient with a parastomal recurrence and a vessel-depleted neck. (*B*) The rib cartilage is removed with care to preserve the posterior perichondrium so as to protect the internal mammary artery and vein during the dissection. (*C*) The internal mammary artery and vein are shown. Distal ligation and caudal rotation of the vessels allows for favorable microvascular anastomosis.

and vein, rather than to compromise on a potentially unreliable vessel so as to avoid further dissection. It is also important for the reconstructive surgeon to have a series of alternative options for recipient vessels, should they be needed in the primary or secondary settings.

FLAP SELECTION

A large number of donor sites are in the armamentarium of the modern reconstructive surgeon. Matching the particular demands of the defect with the appropriate donor tissue(s) is of utmost importance. In a salvage setting, additional considerations should influence flap selection. In our experience, vascularized muscle provides added protection against infection. This principle is well described in the vascular surgery literature in which healthy muscle is often used to increase local tissue oxygen tension, augment the delivery of immune cells and antibiotics, and eliminate dead space.[26] Although vascularized fat may achieve the goal of replacing lost volume, muscle is invaluable for vascular protection in the case of a salivary fistula. When scapular bone is used to reconstruct the mandible following a composite resection of the oral cavity and/or oropharynx, the latissimus dorsi muscle, perfused by the thoracodorsal branch of the subscapular artery, can be harvested and used for coverage of the carotid artery, the jugular vein, and the microvascular pedicle. Anchored superiorly to the reconstructed segment of the mandible, a potential salivary leak is directed superficial to the muscle, effectively protecting the vessels beneath. The authors prefer to use the subscapular system chimeric flap, rather than a fibular free flap, in salvage reconstruction of a composite oral cavity/oropharynx defect (**Fig. 2**).[27] When vascularized muscle is

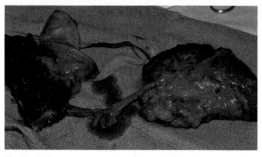

Fig. 2. Subscapular system chimeric flap incorporating scapula bone, parascapular skin paddle, and latissimus dorsi muscle. The length of the thoracodorsal pedicle allows a degree of freedom in manipulating the components of the flap independent from each other in a complex 3-dimensional defect.

not incorporated in the composite flap and brought into the defect as part of the free tissue transfer, we routinely cover the vessels of the neck with a pectoralis major rotational flap. The muscle helps to avoid vessel exposure in case of neck wound break down. This is especially important when the skin cannot be closed without tension, as is often the case with the loss of elasticity associated with radiation exposure. The excess bulk of the muscle can be left exposed, and epithelialization occurs in a matter of weeks. In our experience, acceptable cosmetic results can be expected without the use of skin grafts. Muscle atrophy restores the neck contour to near normal within several months. In chimeric flaps, where all components are supplied by the common vascular pedicle, the exposed muscle can serve an additional role of a flap monitor.

LARYNGOPHARYNGEAL AND ESOPHAGEAL RECONSTRUCTION

Today, primary radiation or chemoradiation treatment of laryngeal and hypopharyngeal squamous cell carcinoma is often the preferred modality. This is largely due to the favorable oncologic and functional outcomes of this organ-preservation strategy in early-stage tumors.[28,29] Failure of nonsurgical modalities to cure the disease or to leave the patient with a functional larynx necessitates salvage surgery in up to 40% of patients.[30] Thus, as the primary treatment shifted toward organ preservation, the demand for reconstruction of salvage-irradiated laryngopharyngeal and pharyngoesophageal defects has increased. The goals of the reconstructive effort should be to effectively separate the respiratory and digestive tracts, avoid exposure of the great vessels and the mediastinal structures to saliva, and to allow for rapid rehabilitation of the swallowing and speech function. Commonly seen complications of pharyngeal reconstruction include a salivary fistula and stenosis of the neopharyngeal lumen.

In patients undergoing salvage total laryngectomy with primary closure, fistula is seen in 34.1% of those with a history of chemoradiation and in 22.8% of patients treated with radiotherapy alone. "Onlay," or flap-reinforced pharyngeal closure, decreases the incidence of a fistula to 10.3%.[31] Where mucosa is insufficient for a tension-free primary closure, a fasciocutaneous or a myocutaneous flap must be inset to recreate the neopharynx. Preservation of even a small strip of pharyngeal mucosa avoids a circumferential scar and reduces the risk of stenosis. Finally, in cases in which a circumferential pharyngectomy defect was created, several options are available to the reconstructive surgeon for reestablishing digestive tract continuity. Tubed forearm free flap has the advantage of introducing thin and pliable tissue into the defect. With the suture line placed anteriorly, the fat and fascia extension of the flap (also known as the "beaver tail"[32]) can be used to cover the vascular pedicle and the great vessels. Effective flap monitoring of this buried reconstruction can be accomplished by incorporating a monitoring skin paddle into the neck suture line (**Fig. 3**). It is critical to avoid stricture at the distal/esophageal anastomosis. The posterior wall of the esophagus can be split longitudinally with a wedge of the cutaneous flap inset into the apex to avoid circumferential stenosis. Additionally, a salivary bypass tube can be placed to stent the lumen open during the healing process. Tight closure over the bypass tube must be avoided, as the pressure on the suture line may interfere with wound healing. Anteriolateral thigh flap can produce comparable results,[33] but is of limited use in patients with unfavorable body habitus often encountered in the Western population. Pectoralis major rotation flap, although often used as a suture line overlay, is not conducive to being tubed given its excessive bulk.

Other options for reconstruction of the pharyngoesophageal segment include enteric flaps such as the gastric pull-up, free jejunum, and the gastro-omental. Gastric pull-up offers a solution for near-total or total esophagectomy defects with a single anastomotic suture line performed through the cervical exposure. This technique, however, is associated with a high perioperative morbidity of 50% and mortality of 8%.[34] Wound-healing complications in previously radiated patients increase the risk of mediastinitis. Jejunal free flap introduces preformed tube with secretory mucosal lining for circumferential pharyngeal reconstruction. The most common complications are the late distal anastomotic stricture, occurring in 11% of cases, and abdominal complications, occurring in 5.8% of cases.[35] The gastro-omental free flap is another option, with well-vascularized omentum facilitating healing in unfavorable wound environments.

Although single-stage reconstruction should be the goal of pharyngoesophageal reconstruction, some patients are poor surgical candidates for free tissue transfer or for intra-abdominal procedures necessary for enteric transpositions. Utilization of local skin flaps in a 2-stage reconstruction, such as a Wookey closure, may afford the best and safest outcome. This technique also may be used when the initial reconstructive effort has failed.

DEAD SPACE

The obliteration of dead space has to be a priority if one is to avoid complications in head and neck reconstruction. Space unfilled with soft tissue is a reservoir for stagnant fluid. Hematomas and seromas reserve potential spaces for infection and abscess formation.[36] In addition, vessels that are not covered by soft tissue are at risk of desiccation or exposure to the erosive environment of saliva and/or pus. This can lead to catastrophic injury to the vessel wall with arterial blow-out, hemorrhage, and death.

As mentioned in the previous section, muscle brought up as part of the free flap, or rotated into the defect from a regional donor site is ideal for coverage of the neck vessels and of the pedicle, as well as for elimination of potential dead space.[37] Whether it is the infratemporal fossa in skull base reconstruction, the parapharyngeal space in oropharyngeal reconstruction, or the upper and posterior neck in oromandibular reconstruction, dead space should be obliterated whenever possible.

Any space that cannot be filled with soft tissue should be adequately drained. Careful planning of drain placement cannot be overemphasized.

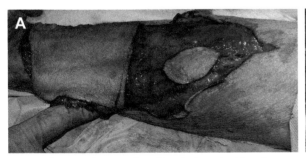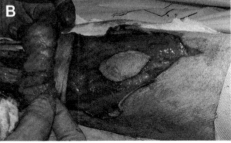

Fig. 3. (*A*) Radial forearm free flap designed with a beaver tail of subcutaneous fat and fascia that supplies a monitoring paddle that is inset in the lateral neck suture line. (*B*) Circumferential pharyngeal defect is repaired by tubing the flap with the suture line placed anteriorly and the beaver tail protecting the vascular pedicle from a potential salivary leak.

The authors prefer passive drainage with Penrose drains. Suction drainage is avoided for fear of negative-pressure injury to the anastomosis. The drain closest to the anastomosis, and deep to the muscle cover, should be removed first to allow healing of the deep surface of the muscle to the tissues of the neck. The drain lateral to the muscle is left in place slightly longer to create a path of least resistance that redirects any potential salivary leak away from the pedicle.

WOUND COMPLICATIONS

Surgical complications will invariably occur in the course of performing reconstructive surgery in the salvage setting in irradiated patients. Effective management of these complications is a measure of experience and careful planning. Wound breakdown and salivary leaks have variable consequences depending on the location in relation to the surrounding structures. They can be categorized into safe and unsafe wounds. A safe wound is any wound that does not compromise the vascular pedicle of the flap and does not expose the carotid artery to infection or desiccation. These range from skin suture line dehiscence over healthy muscle to orocutaneous or pharyngocutaneous fistulas. The first goal is to ensure that a wound does not track to expose the vessels to an adverse environment. If there is a risk that a salivary leak can progress to endanger the vessels of the neck, it must be redirected away using a Penrose or a suction drain. Once the salivary fistula has been redirected for several days and the flaps have seated over the vital structures, packing can be introduced into the wound to promote secondary healing. The closure of the fistula may require new tissue to be introduced into the defect and can be done in a delayed fashion, once the patient's medical condition has been optimized. In the case of safe wounds that do not communicate with the upper aerodigestive tract, active wound debridement using wet to dry packing or negative-pressure wound therapy is usually effective to promote healing by secondary intention. Although wound breakdown is never the goal, a safe wound is not a matter of chance, but rather a product of proper preoperative design and intraoperative execution. Rather than counting on radiated tissues healing, the surgeon should ensure that the critical structures in the neck are protected with well-vascularized tissue. If this is achieved, time is on the surgeon's and the patient's side, and healing by secondary intention often becomes the safest option.

When a wound is not safe or is deemed to be unstable, urgent intervention is required. Infection, or a leak of saliva that affects the pedicle, is associated with a significant risk of thrombosis and flap loss. The proinflammatory state increases risk of clotting in the vessels supplying the flap. Attempts at revision microvascular salvage surgery in this setting are rarely successful. Similarly, long-term exposure of an irradiated carotid artery to saliva weakens the vessel wall, increasing the risk of a life-threatening blow-out. Skin breakdown over a free flap pedicle exposes the vessels to the external environment. Effective packing of the wound is often impossible without risk of compression or injury to the vessels and is not considered an optimal strategy unless the patient is unfit to return to the operating theater. If a wound is left open, there is a high risk of infection or desiccation with clotting of the vascular pedicle. Although flap viability may not be compromised immediately, an unsafe wound should be made safe as soon as possible. Prolonged nutrient vessel exposure to an adverse environment has the potential to lead to catastrophic loss of the entire reconstructive effort.

The steps that have to be taken to salvage an unsafe wound are often the same ones that would be taken in the primary setting to avoid this complication. Careful wound wash out, inspection of the vascular pedicle, vessel coverage with a muscle flap, and redirection of the salivary flow away from the pedicle should be accomplished. The pectoralis major flap is the workhorse flap in this flap salvage situation. Other options include other regional flaps, such as the latissimus dorsi flap, sternocleidomastoid muscle flap, or free tissue transfer. Timely intervention is critical in this scenario and conservative measures are likely to lead to further lost ground.

PLAN B

Although everything should be done to optimize the success of the reconstructive procedure, it is vital to always have a back-up plan. Without this, a failed attempt at reconstruction may leave the patient in a more disadvantageous position, with a worse deformity and suffering. If a flap is to be salvaged after a vascular compromise, the timing of intervention is of the essence. In case of a flap that is fed by more than one artery, or drained by more than one vein, the vessel that is not used in primary anastomosis should be saved as a back-up. For example, when dealing with acute ischemia of the scapula free flap, the subscapular artery used in the initial anastomosis may not be suitable for re-anastomosis in a flap salvage setting. Establishing retrograde flow through angular, thoracodorsal or branch to the serratus arteries allows further reach to the donor artery and may be attempted in an effort to save the flap.

The limiting factor in a second attempt at a reconstruction is commonly the lack of suitable recipient vessels in the neck. It is helpful to know the status of the remaining recipient vasculature before undertaking the reexploration. This status can be defined during the primary reconstruction by taking note of what options remain available at the end of the procedure. This information will certainly provide a degree of reassurance for any surgeon who has the misfortune of "starting from scratch." An alternative donor site can be considered, and the need for arterial or venous grafts anticipated preoperatively. The second attempts after failed initial free tissue transfer are much more challenging, and the cause of the initial failure must be considered carefully to avoid repeating the mistake.[38,39]

SUMMARY

Reconstructive management of patients who are undergoing head and neck ablation for disease persistence or recurrence in a previously irradiated field can be associated with a specific set of challenges. With careful planning and anticipation of potential hurdles, the surgeon and patient can anticipate rates of success similar to those achieved in the primary setting. It is imperative that initiating surgery in this population of patients should be performed only by experienced surgeons who have a multitude of reconstructive techniques at their disposal.

REFERENCES

1. Salemark L. International survey of current microvascular practices in free tissue transfer and replantation surgery. Microsurgery 1991;12:308–11.
2. Eckardt A, Fokas K. Microsurgical reconstruction in the head and neck region: an 18-year experience with 500 consecutive cases. J Craniomaxillofac Surg 2003;31:197–201.
3. Suh JD, Sercarz JA, Abemayor E, et al. Analysis of outcome and complications in 400 cases of microvascular head and neck reconstruction. Arch Otolaryngol Head Neck Surg 2004;130:962–6.
4. Alam DS, Nuara M, Christian J. Analysis of outcomes of vascularized flap reconstruction in patients with advanced mandibular osteoradionecrosis. Otolaryngol Head Neck Surg 2009;141:196–201.
5. Baumann DP, Yu P, Hanasono MM, et al. Free flap reconstruction of osteoradionecrosis of the mandible: a 10-year review and defect classification. Head Neck 2011;33:800–7.
6. Zaghi S, Danesh J, Hendizadeh L, et al. Changing indications for maxillomandibular reconstruction with osseous free flaps: a 17-year experience with 620 consecutive cases at UCLA and the impact of osteoradionecrosis. Laryngoscope 2014;124:1329–35.
7. Deng J, Ridner SH, Dietrich MS, et al. Factors associated with external and internal lymphedema in patients with head-and-neck cancer. Int J Radiat Oncol Biol Phys 2012;84:e319–28.
8. Wang J, Boerma M, Fu Q, et al. Radiation responses in skin and connective tissues: effect on wound healing and surgical outcome. Hernia 2006;10:502–6.
9. Mathes SJ, Alexander J. Radiation injury. Surg Oncol Clin N Am 1996;5:809–24.
10. Wong LY, Wei WI, Lam LK, et al. Salvage of recurrent head and neck squamous cell carcinoma after primary curative surgery. Head Neck 2003;25:953–9.
11. Taki S, Homma A, Oridate N, et al. Salvage surgery for local recurrence after chemoradiotherapy or radiotherapy in hypopharyngeal cancer patients. Eur Arch Otorhinolaryngol 2010;267:1765–9.
12. Röösli C, Studer G, Stoeckli SJ. Salvage treatment for recurrent oropharyngeal squamous cell carcinoma. Head Neck 2010;32:989–96.
13. Schwartz GJ, Mehta RH, Wenig BL, et al. Salvage treatment for recurrent squamous cell carcinoma of the oral cavity. Head Neck 2000;22:34–41.
14. Matoscevic K, Graf N, Pezier TF, et al. Success of salvage treatment a critical appraisal of salvage rates for different subsites of HNSCC. Otolaryngol Head Neck Surg 2014;151(3):454–61.
15. McGregor AD, MacDonald D. Patterns of spread of squamous cell carcinoma to the ramus of the mandible. Head Neck 1993;15:440–4.
16. Wax MK, Bascom DA, Myers LL. Marginal mandibulectomy vs segmental mandibulectomy: indications and controversies. Arch Otolaryngol Head Neck Surg 2002;128:600–3.
17. Choi S, Schwartz DL, Farwell DG, et al. Radiation therapy does not impact local complication rates after free flap reconstruction for head and neck cancer. Arch Otolaryngol Head Neck Surg 2004;130:1308–12.
18. Deutsch M, Kroll SS, Ainsle N, et al. Influence of radiation on late complications in patients with free fibular flaps for mandibular reconstruction. Ann Plast Surg 1999;42:662–4.
19. Bengtson BP, Schusterman MA, Baldwin BJ, et al. Influence of prior radiotherapy on the development of postoperative complications and success of free tissue transfers in head and neck cancer reconstruction. Am J Surg 1993;166:326–30.
20. Kroll SS, Robb GL, Reece GP, et al. Does prior irradiation increase the risk of total or partial free-flap loss? J Reconstr Microsurg 1998;14:263–8.

21. Moreno MA, Skoracki RJ, Hanna EY, et al. Microvascular free flap reconstruction versus palatal obturation for maxillectomy defects. Head Neck 2010;32:860–8.

22. Urken ML, Vickery C, Weinberg H, et al. Geometry of the vascular pedicle in free tissue transfers to the head and neck. Arch Otolaryngol Head Neck Surg 1989;115:954–60.

23. Urken ML, Higgins KM, Lee B, et al. Internal mammary artery and vein: recipient vessels for free tissue transfer to the head and neck in the vessel-depleted neck. Head Neck 2006;28:797–801.

24. Arnez Z, Valdatta L, Tyler M, et al. Anatomy of the internal mammary veins and their use in free TRAM flap breast reconstruction. Br J Plast Surg 1995;48:540–5.

25. Jacobson AS, Eloy JA, Park E, et al. Vessel-depleted neck: techniques for achieving microvascular reconstruction. Head Neck 2008;30:201–7.

26. Seify H, Moyer HR, Jones GE, et al. The role of muscle flaps in wound salvage after vascular graft infections: the Emory experience. Plast Reconstr Surg 2006;117:1325–33.

27. Gibber MJ, Clain JB, Jacobson AS, et al. Subscapular system of flaps: an 8-year experience with 105 patients. Head Neck 2015;37(8):1200–6.

28. Mendenhall WM, Parsons JT, Stringer SP, et al. T1-T2 vocal cord carcinoma: a basis for comparing the results of radiotherapy and surgery. Head Neck Surg 1988;10:373–7.

29. Pellitteri PK, Kennedy TL, Vrabec DP, et al. Radiotherapy: the mainstay in the treatment of early glottic carcinoma. Arch Otolaryngol Head Neck Surg 1991;117:297–301.

30. Ganly I, Patel SG, Matsuo J, et al. Results of surgical salvage after failure of definitive radiation therapy for early-stage squamous cell carcinoma of the glottic larynx. Arch Otolaryngol Head Neck Surg 2006;132:59–66.

31. Sayles M, Grant DG. Preventing pharyngocutaneous fistula in total laryngectomy: a systematic review and meta-analysis. Laryngoscope 2014;124:1150–63.

32. Seikaly H, Rieger J, O'Connell D, et al. Beavertail modification of the radial forearm free flap in base of tongue reconstruction: technique and functional outcomes. Head Neck 2009;31:213–9.

33. Yu P, Robb GL. Pharyngoesophageal reconstruction with the anterolateral thigh flap: a clinical and functional outcomes study. Plast Reconstr Surg 2005;116:1845–55.

34. Surkin MI, Lawson W, Biller HF. Analysis of the methods of pharyngoesophageal reconstruction. Head Neck Surg 1984;6:953–70.

35. Shangold L, Urken M, Lawson W. Jejunal transplantation for pharyngoesophageal reconstruction. Otolaryngol Clin North Am 1991;24:1321–42.

36. Johnson J, Cummings C. Hematoma after head and neck surgery–a major complication? Otolaryngology 1977;86:ORL171–5.

37. Li J, Han Z. Sternocleidomastoid muscle flap used for repairing the dead space after supraomohyoid neck dissection. Int J Clin Exp Med 2015;8:1296.

38. Fearon JA, Cuadros CL, May JW Jr. Flap failure after microvascular free-tissue transfer: the fate of a second attempt. Plast Reconstr Surg 1990;86:746–51.

39. Bozikov K, Arnez Z. Factors predicting free flap complications in head and neck reconstruction. J Plast Reconstr Aesthet Surg 2006;59:737–42.

Unfavorable Results After Free Tissue Transfer to Head and Neck
Lessons Based on Experience from the University of Toronto

Marika Kuuskeri, MD, PhD,
Anne C. O'Neill, MBBCh, MMedSci, FRCS(Plast), MSc, PhD,
Stefan O.P. Hofer, MD, PhD, FRCSC*

KEYWORDS

- Free tissue transfer • Unfavorable result • Oral cavity • Mandible • Maxilla • Facial reconstruction
- Skull base reconstruction

KEY POINTS

- When performing head and neck reconstructions precise knowledge of function and aesthetic requirements of each specific area is mandatory. Careful assessment of what is missing and replacing like with like is essential.
- Development of microsurgical techniques has enabled reconstruction of more complex defects with better functional and aesthetic results.
- Microsurgical techniques have not been able to prevent unfavorable outcomes as they have allowed ablative surgery that was previously not possible due to the lack in reconstructive abilities.
- Functional as well as aesthetic suboptimal results can lead to major impairment of quality of life. The awareness of all possible adverse effects characteristic to each anatomic site is the key to avoiding and managing them.

INTRODUCTION

Head and neck surgery has improved through significant changes and development over the past decades. Factors contributing to this favorable progress include better understanding of anatomy, improved preoperative imaging, more precise delivery of radiation, and advances in surgical technique.[1] Development of microsurgery has enabled reconstruction of virtually any defect after ablative surgery. The foundation for success in head and neck surgery is the restoration of function and aesthetics for which microsurgical reconstruction is often the method of choice. With free tissue transfer, it is possible to replace ablated tissues with similar well-perfused tissues and reconstructions can be individually planned to fulfill the tissue requirements of the defect. Microvascular reconstruction has become a reliable way to recreate ablated tissues, as microvascular success rate is approximately 97% in most high-volume centers.[2–4]

The definition of an acceptable result in head neck surgery has evolved over time. From the earlier simple need to fill the hole, we have advanced to a fuller understanding of the need to

---

Disclosure Statement: Nothing to disclose.
Division of Plastic Surgery, Department of Surgery, University Health Network, University of Toronto, 200 Elizabeth Street, 8N-865, Toronto, Ontario M5G2C4, Canada
* Corresponding author.
E-mail address: Stefan.hofer@uhn.ca

Clin Plastic Surg 43 (2016) 639–651
http://dx.doi.org/10.1016/j.cps.2016.05.003

exactly specify the defect and missing components. In reconstructing the form and function of the ablated tissues, failure to appreciate the unique features of individual tissues will most likely lead to suboptimal outcome.[5] Unfavorable results in head and neck free flap surgery are more than just a failed flap but also include cases in which reasonable restoration or acceptable aesthetics have not been achieved. In addition, an unfavorable result has been obtained if unacceptable donor site morbidity or patient dissatisfaction is present.

The purpose of the current article is to provide an overview of the functional and aesthetic unfavorable results of head and neck reconstruction, and provide suggestions on how to address these issues. Understanding the consequences of an unsuccessful reconstruction provides the foundation for proper planning and personalized approach to reconstruction of lost structures.

UNFAVORABLE RESULTS IN ORAL CAVITY RECONSTRUCTION

The oral cavity is composed of the floor of the mouth, the anterior two-thirds of the tongue, buccal mucosa, hard palate, mandibular and maxillary alveolar ridges, and retromolar trigones. The oral cavity is bordered by the lips anteriorly, and the base of the tongue and soft palate posteriorly. All these different structures have unique properties that will be affected by ablative surgery. These properties include important roles in speech, taste, and mastication. The structures of the oral cavity are also used for breathing, facial expressions, and social interactions. Partial resection of many of these functional structures is frequently required to achieve disease control.[5] An unfavorable result in oral cavity reconstruction is more often a problem of function than aesthetics. Speech can become unintelligible and impair social life. Also, ability to chew and swallow food can be severely affected. Suboptimal results can have serious effects on the patient's quality of life.

Floor of Mouth

When planning a reconstruction of the floor of the mouth, it is important to acknowledge that no one part can be reconstructed without it having an effect on the other parts. The main issues in designing the reconstruction are restoring the buccogingival and/or labiogingival sulcus of adequate depth, avoiding excessive height of the floor of the mouth, and allowing optimal tongue mobility by restoring exactly what has been removed.[5] Major indications for floor of the mouth flap

reconstruction are to close defects that communicate with the neck to prevent vascular blow out caused by salivary contamination of the major vessels, and to achieve coverage of exposed mandibular bone which may not remucosalize spontaneously especially in the setting of radiation therapy.[6]

The precise planning and careful analysis of what is missing will prevent the reconstruction with a flap that is either too small or too large. In either condition, with excessive bulk or too much tension, the mobility of the tongue is affected, having a significant impact on both the speech and swallowing. This emphasizes the importance of using a flap of adequate thickness. The radial forearm flap is still the most popular flap when a thin reconstruction of the floor of the mouth is needed, although the anterolateral thigh flap has gained increasing popularity.[7] One option is to reconstruct a floor of the mouth defect with a fascial or muscle flap and let it reepithelialize by the surrounding mucosal surface. These non–skin bearing flaps can be subject to considerable contraction as a result of wound-healing forces. In the presence of radiation, remucosalization may not occur.[5] Xerostomia following radiation is a common problem and jejunal patches and colon patches have been used for floor of the mouth reconstruction in an attempt to address this debilitating condition. Although these flaps are thin and have the ability to produce mucus, the risk of donor site morbidity and limited ability to endure radiation have prevented them from being widely used.[1]

In the case of an unsatisfactory result after reconstruction, revision may become necessary. The second procedure is typically required to reduce bulkiness or add tissue to gain mobility or depth. When performing de-bulking, one must beware of creating too much tension on tissues or exposing intraoral bone. If the sulcus is too shallow or the tongue movement is limited, additional tissue needs to be brought in. This can range from a full-thickness skin graft to local flaps or even a new free flap (**Fig. 1**). Sometimes simple release of scar tissue will improve movement of the tongue, but careful patient selection is critical, as in some cases this release will diminish the function of the tongue, as remaining tongue function can be dependent on the fixed less-mobile position (**Box 1**).[5]

Tongue

The tongue has a highly specialized function and reconstruction can be challenging. The aim of the reconstruction is to restore and/or maintain the

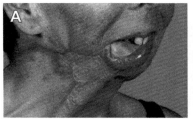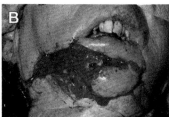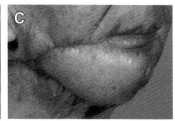

Fig. 1. (*A*) Patient with bulky floor of mouth reconstruction obliterating the labiogingival sulcus complicated by external skin loss that was reconstructed with a split-thickness skin graft at the time of ablative surgery. The split-thickness skin graft causes additional contraction resulting in downward pull of the lip. The outcome of this initial reconstruction can be scored as 100% flap survival with complete functional and aesthetic failure. (*B*) Revision surgery is directed at removal of the split-thickness skin graft that caused contraction and full release of the scarred tissues to restore lower lip position and thus addressing complete oral incontinence. Reconstructive requirement is for a free flap, as the radiated tissue bed requires well-vascularized tissue transfer to allow healing. (*C*) An anterolateral thigh free flap was used to provide well-vascularized tissue for permanent restoration of lip position. The labiogingival sulcus was debulked at the same operation. A permanent result with normal oral continence was maintained at follow-up after 1 year.

important roles in speech, swallowing, and airway protection. Tongue reconstruction is focused on preservation of optimal mobility. After tongue reconstruction, the tongue should be able to contact the hard palate for speech articulation, and to clear the oral cavity and move food and secretions from anterior to posterior.[8,9]

Smaller defects can be closed primarily. Tongue tissue should not be used to close adjacent defects as this will significantly impair mobility.[5] Larger defects that involve around half of the tongue will mostly require a free flap for reconstruction. Mostly a thin pliable flap, such as a radial forearm or thin anterolateral thigh flap, will preserve the mobility of the tongue (**Fig. 2**). It is important to ensure that sufficient bulk remains to obliterate the oral cavity space when the mouth

is closed, and to prevent secretions from directly draining to the larynx.[1] The approach for reconstruction of total or near-total glossectomy defects is slightly different. Bulkier flaps are needed to replace the resected volume. Larger flaps can provide better bulk so as to assist in swallowing. Still, patients with total glossectomy are at high risk of remaining dependent on parenteral nutrition and may suffer from frequent episodes of aspiration. When considering the location of the defect on the tongue, it can be generally stated that anterior and lateral tongue defects often have limited requirement for bulk and can be reconstructed with thinner flaps, whereas more posterior defects require more bulk.[5]

Revision surgery following tongue reconstruction may be required to improve functional outcome. As mentioned previously, there are 2 goals of these secondary procedures: to improve movement or reduce bulkiness. In the pursuit of better mobility skin grafts, local flaps or even free flaps might be needed. The reduction of bulkiness is more straightforward, but the improvement of function is often less than expected or desired (**Box 2**).[5]

Palate

The palate forms the roof of the mouth and it separates the oral cavity from the nasal cavity. The palate is divided into anterior bony hard palate and posterior muscular soft palate. The functional importance of the hard palate lies in speech. The mobile soft palate is involved in swallowing, breathing, and speech. During swallowing and speech, the soft palate separates the oral from the nasal cavity. After resection, reconstructive challenges arise from these functional requirements. An open connection between the nasal

---

Box 1
Floor of mouth reconstruction

- Goal:
  - Watertight closure of oral cavity from neck
- Salient points:
  - Avoid excessive bulk or tightness to preserve tongue mobility
  - Preserve bucco/labiogingival sulcus to prevent oral incontinence
- In case of an unfavorable result:
  - Excision of excess bulk
  - Addition of new tissue to resolve tightness
- Cave:
  - Radiated local tissues can give poor healing and revision can give bigger problems

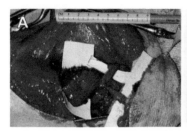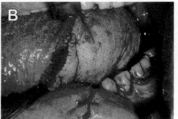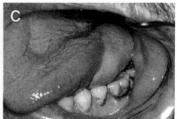

Fig. 2. (*A*) A thin anterolateral thigh flap can be used for lateral tongue defects. In this flap elevation, a small segment of vastus lateralis muscle is included to add bulk to the base of tongue that has partially been resected. The main perforator can be seen with a small block of muscle on a side branch of the perforator. (*B*) The intraoperative view shows a tidy inset restoring proper volume of the tongue. (*C*) At 1 year after operation, the anterolateral thigh flap has incorporated well into the native tongue. The tongue has maintained excellent mobility.

and oral cavities will result in open nasal speech and oral intake escaping through the nose.

Midpalatal resections that spare all the teeth, premaxillary resections that include only the incisors, and unilateral posterior defects that involve only the teeth posterior to the canine may be suitable to be treated by an obturator prosthetic. Smaller defects also can be reconstructed with local flaps from adjacent palatal mucosa or tongue. However, in ablative cancer surgery, a free flap often will be required.[5] Defects involving 50% or more of the palate usually require free flap reconstruction, partly due to the lack of supporting tissues to stabilize the prosthesis.[1] There are studies supporting the opinion that even in small or medium-size defects, a free flap reconstruction provides superior results compared with a prosthetic device by improving patients' daily quality of life.[10–12] For free flaps, the reconstruction with soft tissue flaps will generally give a good result.

When reconstructing soft palate, there are 2 main considerations. First, oral and nasal cavities need to be kept separate, and second, there needs to be sufficient bulk in the back of the oral cavity for the tongue to push against for swallowing. For smaller defects, a radial forearm flap is sufficient. It should be folded so that both the nasal and oral surfaces are reconstructed. If the nasal surface is left raw, the flap will shrink significantly due to wound-healing forces, and the shrinkage is even more pronounced in the presence of radiation therapy. For larger defects, a bulkier flap, such as an anterolateral thigh flap, is indicated to provide sufficient volume for adequate postoperative swallowing (**Fig. 3**). All flaps used to reconstruct the soft palate should be planned so that they reach close to or touch the posterior pharyngeal wall, because they will experience considerable postoperative shrinkage due to the lack of surrounding support, which is normally present in the hard palate but not the soft palate.[5]

In the event of a suboptimal result after the primary reconstruction of hard palate there are usually 2 complaints: leakage of oral intake through the nose or unintelligible open nasal speech. If after soft palate reconstruction the patient suffers from the open nasal speech, this condition may be improved with a cranially or caudally based pharyngoplasty (**Box 3**).

UNFAVORABLE RESULTS IN MANDIBLE RECONSTRUCTION

From a functional point of view, mandible reconstruction needs to maintain the framework to support the anterior oral cavity and neck structures, enable mastication, provide the basis for dental rehabilitation, preserve maximal mouth opening, and maintain proper occlusion.[5,6] With reconstruction, the exact contour should be restored, as a change in the arc size will result in malocclusion for dentulous patients. Adequate bone height is essential when planning implant-based dental rehabilitation.[5] From an aesthetic standpoint,

---

Box 2
Tongue reconstruction

- Goal:
  - Maintain or restore maximal mobility
- Salient points:
  - Mobile tongue defects require less bulk
  - Loss of base of tongue will in general require bulk to allow swallowing
- In case of an unfavorable result:
  - Bulk reduction or release of tethering may improve mobility
- Cave:
  - Revision for limited mobility gives often only very modest improvement at best

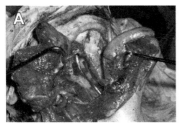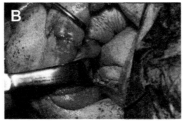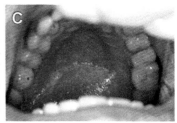

Fig. 3. (A) A large combined hard and soft palate defect is visible through a mandibular split approach. Reconstruction of the defect is with a soft tissue flap, as the remaining hard palate provides sufficient support. The large soft palate resection requires a bulky reconstruction to provide sufficient tissue to enable separation of the oral and nasal cavities. (B) A very large anterolateral thigh flap is inset into the defect. Inset is challenging due to the bulk during surgery. Bulk will decrease in the postoperative period as part of general decrease of swelling. The anterolateral thigh flap will retain significant bulk, as it is a skin and subcutaneous tissue flap as opposed to a muscle flap that loses a large amount of the volume not only as a result of postoperative decrease of swelling but also as a result of muscle atrophy. (C) At 18 months after surgery, the anterolateral has fully integrated into the surrounding palate tissues. Permanent separation of oral and nasal cavity has been achieved. The patient had mild nasal speech after this reconstruction.

preservation of chin height and projection as well as retaining symmetry are main goals.[6]

The classification system for segmental mandibular defects described by Boyd and colleagues[14] is especially useful when planning mandible reconstruction. It describes defects as central (c, including all 4 incisors and 2 canines), lateral (l, condyle is preserved), and hemi-mandible defect (h, lateral defects including the condyle). It also classifies the soft tissue involvement as skin (s), mucosa (m), and no soft tissue involvement (o).[13,14] All these components have an effect on flap selection. Osteocutaneous free flaps are considered the gold standard for segmental mandible reconstruction due to their lower complication rate and ability to restore the mandible to the original state.[6] The fibula flap remains the workhorse flap, as it can provide more than 20 cm of bicortical bone with excellent blood supply and good pedicle length.[13] Because of the dual periosteal and endosteal blood supply multiple osteotomies can be performed as close as 2 cm apart without concern for bone viability. Central mandibular defects require osseous flaps to prevent airway collapse, oral incontinence, and facial distortion. Lateral defects can also be reconstructed with soft tissue only in selected edentulous patients.[5,6] Early postoperative mobilization of the reconstructed area is recommended to prevent trismus.

Unfavorable results after osteocutaneous free flap mandibular reconstruction include excessive soft tissue bulk transferred with the bone flap, osteoradionecrosis following postoperative radiation, failure of the bony reconstruction in the central defect causing total collapse of the remaining mandible, and trismus. Excessive soft tissue in mandibular reconstruction will prevent dental rehabilitation. Failure to enable dental rehabilitation affects both functional and aesthetic outcomes, as dentures provide important support for the lower lip.[5]

Revision procedures vary from simple debulking to a new free flap. Gingivoplasty techniques might be needed to deepen the buccogingival sulcus. If secondary bone revision surgery is required, this can result in osteoradionecrosis after radiation (**Box 4**, **Fig. 4**).

Box 3
Palate reconstruction

- Goal:
  - Keep the nasal and oral cavities separated
- Salient points:
  - Hard palate defects may be treated by an obturator or small soft tissue flap
  - Soft palate defects need to have sufficient bulk to touch the posterior pharyngeal wall and prevent air leakage.
- In case of an unfavorable result:
  - A pharyngeal flap can be added to improve function after soft palate reconstruction
  - Nasal side lining should be provided to prevent excessive shrinking of a soft tissue flap without any other support
- Cave:
  - The soft palate is muscular, which usually cannot be reconstructed adequately in a cancer-ablative reconstruction followed by radiation

Box 4
Mandible reconstruction

- Goal:
  - Create framework support for oral cavity and allow occlusion
- Salient points:
  - Segmental defects will usually require an osteocutaneous flap
  - Lateral defects may be reconstructed with soft tissue only in edentulous patients. This may cause some drift of remaining mandible
- In case of an unfavorable result:
  - Gingivoplasty techniques to reduce bulk may be required
- Cave:
  - Bone reconstruction needs to be done very meticulously, as revision after radiation can cause osteoradionecrosis

UNFAVORABLE RESULTS IN MAXILLA RECONSTRUCTION

The defect resulting from maxillary resection has considerable effect on both aesthetics and function. The paired maxillary bones are pivotal structures, forming the skeletal foundation of the midface. The goals of maxillary reconstruction are to restore dimensions of the face (height, width, projection), separate the orbit and oral cavity from the sinonasal complex, support the globe, provide a foundation for dental rehabilitation, and maintain oral competence, speech, and deglutition.[6,15] The midface is the area in which reconstructive techniques continue to evolve.[1]

A useful algorithm to help in planning midface reconstruction is based on reconstructing the 6 walls of the maxillary bones.[16] These walls are surrounded by the orbit above, the cheek anteriorly and laterally, the nasal cavity medially, the skull base posteriorly, and oral cavity inferiorly. According to the algorithm, type I defects (limited anterior and medial wall defects, no palatal involvement) can be reconstructed with fasciocutaneous free flaps. For type II defects (subtotal maxillectomy, resection of lower 5 walls, but not orbital floor), an osteocutaneous flap is needed to restore palatal competence and bony support for dental rehabilitation. In type IIIa defects in which all 6 maxillary walls are resected (total maxillectomy with preservation of the orbit) the reconstruction becomes complex. The orbital wall must be reconstructed precisely to support the globe. Inaccurate correction will result in impaired vision, which can be difficult to correct, especially in the setting of radiation.[15,17] In IIIb defects (total maxillectomy with orbital exenteration) a bulky flap with multiple skin island is preferred. Also for type IV defects, which include the upper 5 maxillary walls and orbit, leaving the dura and brain exposed (orbitomaxillectomy with preservation of the palate), a similar free flap forms a good option[6,13,16] (**Fig. 5**).

Unfavorable results can occur when, following resection of the anterior maxillary arch, a soft tissue flap alone is used for reconstruction, resulting in the loss of midfacial projection, lack of stable surface for mastication, and inability to provide the patient with osseointegrated implants. An osseous flap such as the fibula free flap presents an excellent option with well-vascularized bicortical bone that may easily be osteotomized and individually tailored to fit virtually any osseous defect of the midface.[18] Muscle flaps are excellent options when the orbit is exenterated, but they are

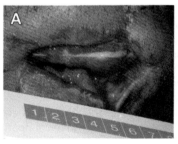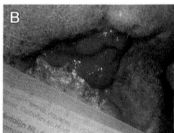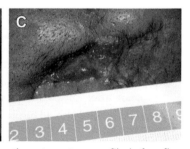

Fig. 4. (*A*) Skin breakdown at 2 weeks in a previously irradiated neck shows the osteocutaneous fibula free flap, performed for a pathologic fracture as a result of osteoradionecrosis, with the plate in the upper medial corner of the wound slightly exposed. It was decided to manage this breakdown with hyperbaric oxygen treatment and conservative wound management. (*B*) Improvement of the wound was seen after 3 weeks of hyperbaric oxygen evidenced by active hypergranulation, which was managed conservatively. (*C*) From the last available photograph at 6 weeks, the patient continued to heal uneventfully without further breakdown and full fibula flap consolidation remaining so after 4-year follow-up.

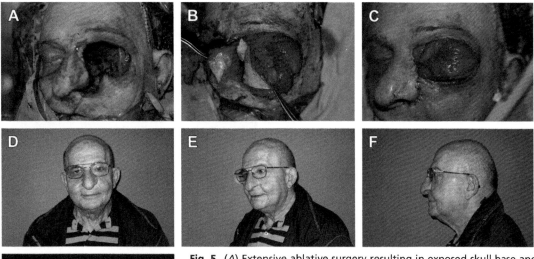

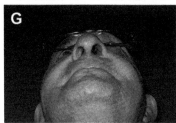

Fig. 5. (A) Extensive ablative surgery resulting in exposed skull base and subtotal maxillectomy with intact palate. (B) A vertical rectus abdominis musculocutaneous flap with a skin paddle to restore inner nasal lining and septal replacement is performed to obliterate the cavity and cover the base of the skull. (C) A very bulky muscle component was covered with a split-thickness skin graft at the end of the operation. The expectation for the flap was to shrink due to postoperative decrease in general swelling as well as muscle atrophy. (D–G) At almost 2 years after surgery without further revision surgery the patient functions well with the use of a facial prosthetic.

rarely ideal when the orbital contents are preserved.[19] As the transferred muscle atrophies over time, volume loss will lead to orbital dystopia, diplopia, and midface flattening.[18,20]

Secondary revision following maxilla reconstruction can address bone and soft tissue augmentation. Solutions may range from fat and bone grafting to second free flaps consisting of only soft tissues and/or bone. Prosthetic rehabilitation is also well developed following maxillary resection (**Box 5**).

UNFAVORABLE RESULTS IN FACIAL RECONSTRUCTION

Reconstruction of the face is based on aesthetic facial zones. The lines between convex and concave surfaces on the face, where light and shadow create visual borders, separate these zones. Larger aesthetic facial units, such as nose and lips, are subdivided into subunits to further refine facial reconstruction. Scars are preferentially placed where these units border to make them less conspicuous.[5,21,22]

In planning facial reconstruction, meticulous analysis of what is missing and what needs to be replaced is required. Quality of tissues needed and demand for structural support of those tissues

requires careful design. Often more than 1 surgery is needed to achieve a satisfactory result.[5]

Facial reconstruction is preferentially performed with local tissues, as this provides better color

---

Box 5
Maxilla reconstruction

- Goal:
  - Maintain or restore midface support on several levels
- Salient points:
  - Defect analysis is paramount to make a proper plan for these highly complex defects
  - Prosthetic rehabilitation is a valuable adjunct to enhance reconstructive outcomes
- In case of an unfavorable result:
  - Soft tissue and/or bone enhancement can be performed in addition to prosthetic rehabilitation
- Cave:
  - Well-vascularized tissue needs to keep all cavities and structures separated, covered and supported.

match and tissue thickness compared with distant free flaps (**Figs. 6** and **7**). In special circumstances, free flap reconstruction of the face will be necessary. On the other hand, scalp reconstruction is more readily amenable to free flap reconstruction providing satisfactory results.

Forehead and Scalp

The use of microvascular techniques has allowed the reconstruction of more complicated and extensive defects of the scalp/forehead area. The aim of the forehead and scalp reconstruction is to cover exposed skull bone and/or contents. The indications for free flap repair in the scalp include previously failed local flaps or their insufficient size, previously applied radiation therapy on a wound bed with exposed bone, most full-thickness calvarial bone loss, and anticipated high-dose radiation therapy.[18,23,24] In the oncological setting, a free flap reconstruction is also the most reliable solution, allowing the patient to proceed with adjuvant therapy with the best wound-healing capacity, and least risk of cerebrospinal fluid leak and infection.[15]

Flap selection for scalp reconstruction has traditionally been for muscle flaps with skin graft. These flaps give a nice contour once they shrink over the skull as the muscle atrophies (**Fig. 8**). Some reconstructive surgeons prefer skin and subcutaneous flaps, as the muscle in some cases can atrophy quite significantly giving rise to recurrent areas of skin graft breakdown.

The main aesthetic concerns of free flap scalp reconstruction are excessive bulk or too thin coverage longer term, incorrect skin color, and lack of hair. Musculocutaneous or thicker cutaneous flaps can result in excessive bulk (**Fig. 9**). This can be corrected by excising the skin paddle of the musculocutaneous flap with skin grafting of the underlying muscle. For thicker cutaneous

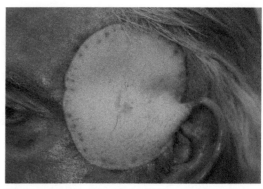

Fig. 7. An anterolateral thigh flap to the temporal area gives good contour but poor color match.

flaps, partial resection or liposuction of the subcutaneous fat of a bulky flap can be performed. Skin areas that are primarily protected from the sun by clothes are unpredictable in the way they will color after they have been transferred to the facial area. When using skin grafts for forehead reconstruction, the best color match may be achieved with grafts taken from the scalp. For scalp reconstruction, the color is often less important because it will be mostly often covered with a hairpiece or wig. Surgical solutions to missing hair are hair transplantation and tissue expansion to cover the bald area in case of more limited hair loss. Simpler, nonsurgical ways to address these issues include hairpieces, wigs, or tattooing in cases of missing eyebrows.[5]

Nose

As a central part of the face, the nose attracts the eye first and therefore cosmetically pleasing reconstruction is essential. Nasal reconstruction follows the 3-layer principle in which inner mucosal lining, osteocartilaginous structural support, and outer skin lining are reconstructed separately. The workhorse flap for nasal reconstruction is the forehead flap. Microvascular distant flaps are used only if other options are unavailable. A free flap can supply nasal lining, while the outer skin will still be reconstructed with a forehead flap for better color match.[25]

Perioral Area and Lips

The lips also have a central role in the aesthetics of the face. The perioral region consists of 5 aesthetic subunits: philtrum, right cutaneous upper lip, left cutaneous upper lip, vermilion, and cutaneous lower lip, which are taken into consideration when planning the reconstruction. The goals of the reconstruction are to retain oral function, competence, and shape. Innervation, sensation, and final cosmesis complete the end result.[26] Lip

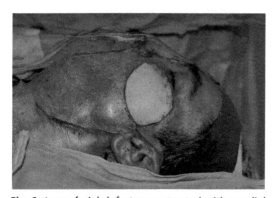

Fig. 6. Large facial defect reconstructed with a radial forearm free flap gives good early contour but poor color match.

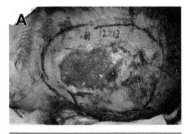
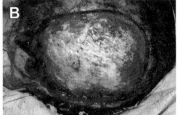
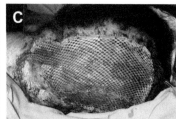
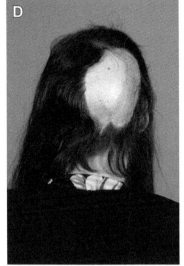
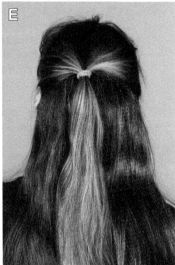

Fig. 8. (*A*) Large basal cell skin cancer of the posterior scalp in a young woman requiring a 12 × 12-cm full-thickness scalp resection. (*B*) Extensive resection defect with additional burring of the external table of the skull. (*C*) At the end of the operation, a large latissimus dorsi free flap with a split-thickness skin graft gives a well-vascularized reconstruction of this extensive defect. (*D*) After 2 years, a nice smooth surface is the end result of the reconstruction. This area is non–hair bearing but allows native hair or a hairpiece to provide inconspicuous cover. (*E*) In this patient with long hair, no further corrections are needed as her own hair covers the area without concern.

reconstruction is mostly performed with local perioral flaps. Free flaps are considered in subtotal or total upper and/or lower lip loss. Traditionally the most common free flap for lip/perioral reconstruction has been the radial forearm flap with incorporation of the palmaris longus tendon to provide lower lip support[27] (**Fig. 10**). Another microsurgical flap option for the perioral area is the gracilis muscle free flap, which can be transferred with a long strip of fascia lata to be used as a supportive structure.[26]

The complications of total or subtotal lip reconstruction are hypertrophic scarring, disfigurement, loss of sensation, microstomia, loss of oral competence, and loss of the natural gingivobuccal sulcus, making the use of dentures difficult.[26,28,29] For microstomia, splints can be useful. A low or obliterated gingivobuccal sulcus can be corrected with local flaps or a skin graft. Many of these problems are difficult to correct secondarily, and therefore careful planning of the primary reconstruction is critical to avoid or minimize these issues.

Periorbital Area

Goals of periorbital reconstruction are preservation of function and position of the globe or prosthesis within the orbit.[30] Periorbital defects can

generally be reconstructed with skin grafts or local tissue rearrangements.[13] When large or composite defects are reconstructed, free tissue transfer is a reliable option. The free flap will obliterate the orbital exenteration defect covering the skull base. In cases of orbital exenteration, it is important to determine whether the patient will use an eye patch or prosthesis. A thin soft tissue coverage should be used if an osseointegrated prosthesis is selected so as to provide a tight seal around the bony support, and to allow enough space for the prosthesis.[15] If an eye patch is selected, a bulkier flap should be selected to fill the cavity and avoid the disfiguring look of an empty socket when the eye patch is removed.

Incorrect flap selection to the orbital socket may make fitting a prosthesis impossible. Excessive bulk of flaps can be addressed by debulking (**Fig. 11**). Volume loss in flaps due to either muscle atrophy or radiation can be corrected by single or sequential lipofilling or in very rare cases by a new free flap reconstruction (**Box 6**).

UNFAVORABLE RESULTS IN SKULL BASE RECONSTRUCTION

The skull base is formed by the anterior, middle, and posterior cranial fossae intracranially. For

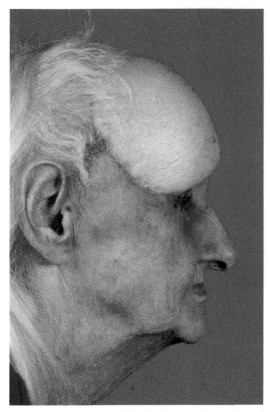

Fig. 9. An anterolateral thigh flap on the scalp will generally not match the skin scalp skin and give an aesthetically poor result.

reconstructive purposes, Irish and colleagues[31] described a 3-region classification system based on tumor anatomic location, tumor growth patterns, and surgical approach. Region I tumors arise from the sinuses, orbit, maxilla, maxillary antrum, midfacial skin, and other local anterior structures and extend to the anterior cranial fossa. Tumors arising from or extending down the clivus to the foramen magnum are also included in region I, because they are also approached anteriorly and behave like anterior skull base tumors. Region I defects usually involve an anterior base of skull bony defect, a dural defect, a varying size dead space from maxillectomy with or without orbital exenteration, a loss of nasal mucosa, and a loss of external skin. Requirements for the reconstruction are reliable dural repair, a flap to fill the dead space, sufficient mucosa, and skin coverage. Bone defects in the skull base do not usually require bone reconstruction, and in most instances can be adequately supported by the soft tissues. Region II tumors arise laterally and primarily involve the infratemporal and pterygopalatine fossa with extension into the middle cranial fossa. Region II tumors have the highest risk of dural involvement compared with regions I and III. Region III tumors arise from within or around temporal bone, including the ear and parotid, with intracranial extension to involve the posterior cranial fossa or middle cranial fossa. Regions II and

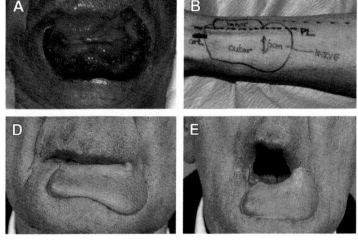

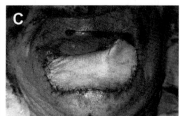

Fig. 10. (A) A near-total lower lip defect with extension into the left upper lip and resection of the left commissure in a middle-aged man. (B) A radial forearm free flap is designed with an inner and outer lining portion of forearm skin and the palmaris longus tendon (PL) in-between to provide support for the lower lip reconstruction. A sensate nerve is included to provide sensation to the lip reconstruction. (C) The intraoperative result of the lower lip reconstruction after microneurovascular anastomoses and skin inset. The PL tendon has already been inset into the right commissure and is about to be woven into and inset into the orbicularis oris musculature of the upper lip. Care is taken to set the tendon at a slightly excessive tension to allow for postoperative loosening. (D) Color and contour of the radial forearm in the face at the potion of the lip is not optimal. Patient was not motivated to have any surgery for contour improvement. (E) Functional outcome was excellent with full oral continence, reasonable mouth opening. and excellent sensation. Sensation in the lower lip is important, as recurrent trauma during eating hot food is a risk.

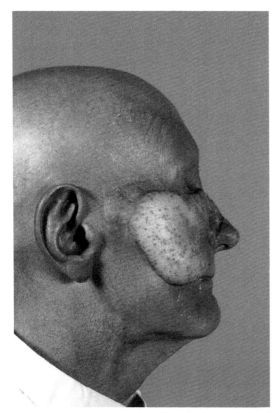

Fig. 11. Fasciocutaneous free flaps in the periorbital area, such as this anterolateral thigh flap after radiation often give bulk issues. The very thin periorbital tissues do not require massive bulk in general. Even a complete orbital exenteration as in this patient will not often result in a massive tissue requirement.

abscess. To prevent infection in this special location, prophylactic antibiotics are usually administered. The risk for cerebrospinal fluid leak and infection can also be diminished with well-vascularized free flap obliteration of dead space and coverage of the exposed areas (**Box 7**).

III skull base resections can also result in bone and dura defects. Skin loss tends to be more extensive, but the amount of soft tissue or dead space tends to be less.[31,32]

Free tissue transfer has had significant impact on the reconstruction of skull base defects. Use of microsurgical techniques has enabled safe reconstruction of defects in which intracranial contents are exposed to the aerodigestive tract.[1] Specific goals in this area are watertight dural repair, separation of the central nervous system from the nasopharynx, obliteration of dead space, reestablishment of orbital and oral cavities, and restoration of facial symmetry and appearance.[32] The reconstruction focuses on prevention of life-threatening central nervous system complications.

The most common complication related to skull base reconstruction is wound infection. These infections require early intervention to avoid fatal central nervous system complications such as cerebrospinal fluid leak, meningitis or intracranial

Box 8
Second free tissue transfer in head and neck reconstruction

- Goal:
  - ○ Salvage a potentially life-threatening condition
  - ○ Enable adjuvant therapy without delay in selected patients
- Salient points:
  - ○ A second free flap after a successful first free flap is a safe procedure
  - ○ A second free flap after a failed first free flap is at higher risk for failure, especially if no clear reason for failure is present
- In case of an unfavorable result:
  - ○ A second free flap is indicated if no other reasonable option is present
- Cave:
  - ○ Intrinsic patient factors need to be considered if a free flap fails without clear cause before a second free flap is performed

SECOND FREE TISSUE TRANSFER IN HEAD AND NECK RECONSTRUCTION

Free tissue transfer offers a safe reconstructive method with mostly manageable complications. Sometimes a second free flap is required to correct treatment-related complications. Ross and colleagues[33] reported that patients who required a second free flap following a previously successful first free flap, for local tumor recurrence, a new second tumor or later complications, such as osteoradionecrosis or plate fracture, showed a free flap success rate of 96%. It is important to recognize, however, that this patient group differs from those requiring a second free flap during the same admission due to failure of the first flap. The success rate in this salvage group was significantly lower at 73% (**Box 8**).

SUMMARY

Development of reconstructive microsurgery has played a pivotal role in management of head and neck cancer. It has enabled resection and safe reconstruction of complex soft tissue and bony defects that would have been otherwise impossible to perform. Free tissue transfer provides reliable, well-vascularized tissue that can be customized to fit any defect size or location. Unfavorable results can be prevented by evaluation of the anatomic site of the cancer and anticipated size and anatomy of defect, assessment of possible donor sites, and evaluation of the need for adjuvant therapies so as to restore the loss of form and function.

REFERENCES

1. Neligan PC. Head and neck reconstruction. Plast Reconstr Surg 2013;131:260–9.
2. Blackwell KE. Unsurpassed reliability of free flaps for head and neck reconstruction. Arch Otolaryngol Head Neck Surg 1999;125:295–9.
3. Frederick JW, Sweeny L, Carroll WR, et al. Outcomes in head and neck reconstruction by surgical site and donor site. Laryngoscope 2013;123: 1612–7.
4. Nuara MJ, Sauder CL, Alam DS. Prospective analysis of outcomes and complications of 300 consecutive microvascular reconstructions. Arch Facial Plast Surg 2009;11:235–9.
5. Hofer SOP, Payne CE. Functional and aesthetic outcome enhancement of head and neck reconstruction through secondary procedures. Semin Plast Surg 2010;24:309–18.
6. Hanasono MM, Matros E, Disa JJ. Important aspects of head and neck reconstruction. Plast Reconstr Surg 2014;134:968–80.
7. Markey J, Knott PD, Fritz MA, et al. Recent advances in head and neck free tissue transfer. Curr Opin Otolaryngol Head Neck Surg 2015;23: 297–301.
8. Chepeha DB, Teknos TN, Shargodorsky J, et al. Rectangle tongue template for reconstruction of the hemiglossectomy defect. Arch Otolaryngol Head Neck Surg 2008;134:993–8.
9. Hsiao HT, Leu YS, Liu CJ, et al. Radial forearm versus anterolateral thigh flap reconstruction after hemiglossectomy: functional assessment of swallowing and speech. J Reconstr Microsurg 2008;24: 85–8.
10. Genden EM, Wallace DI, Okay D, et al. Reconstruction of the hard palate using the radial forearm free flap: indications and outcomes. Head Neck 2004; 26:808–14.
11. Kornblith AB, Zlotolow IM, Gooen J, et al. Quality of life of maxillectomy patients using an obturator prosthesis. Head Neck 1996;18:323–34.
12. Rogers SN, Lowe D, McNally D, et al. Health-related quality of life after maxillectomy: a comparison between prosthetic obturation and free flap. J Oral Maxillofac Surg 2003;61:174–81.
13. Patel SA, Chang EI. Principles and practice of reconstructive surgery for head and neck cancer. Surg Oncol Clin N Am 2015;24:473–89.
14. Boyd JB, Gullane PJ, Rotstein LE, et al. Classification of mandibular defects. Plast Reconstr Surg 1993;92:1266–75.

15. Wei FC, Dayan JH. Scalp, skull, orbit, and maxilla reconstruction and hair transplantation. Plast Reconstr Surg 2013;131:411–24.

16. Cordeiro PG, Santamaria E. A classification system and algorithm for reconstruction of maxillectomy and midfacial defects. Plast Reconstr Surg 2000; 105:2331–46.

17. McCarthy CM, Cordeiro PG. Microvascular reconstruction of oncologic defects of the midface. Plast Reconstr Surg 2010;126:1947–59.

18. Cannady SB, Rosenthal EL, Knott D, et al. Free tissue transfer for head and neck reconstruction. A contemporary review. JAMA Facial Plast Surg 2014;16:367–73.

19. Cordeiro PG, Chen CM. A 15-year review of midface reconstruction after total and subtotal maxillectomy, I: algorithm and outcomes. Plast Reconstr Surg 2012;129:124–36.

20. Le QT, Fu KK, Kaplan M, et al. Treatment of maxillary sinus carcinoma: a comparison of the 1997 and 1977 American Joint Committee on Cancer staging systems. Cancer 1999;86:1700–11.

21. Menick FJ. Facial reconstruction with local and distant tissue: the interface of aesthetic and reconstructive surgery. Plast Reconstr Surg 1998;102: 1424–33.

22. Miller GD, Anstee EJ, Snell JA. Successful replantation of an avulsed scalp by microvascular anastomoses. Plast Reconstr Surg 1976;58:133–6.

23. Hussussian CJ, Reece GP. Microsurgical scalp reconstruction in the patient with cancer. Plast Reconstr Surg 2002;109:1828–34.

24. Chang KP, Lai CH, Chang CH, et al. Free flap options for reconstruction of complicated scalp and calvarial defects: report of a series of cases and literature review. Microsurgery 2010;30:13–8.

25. Menick FJ. Nasal reconstruction. Plast Reconstr Surg 2010;125:138–50.

26. Anvar BA, Evans BCD, Evans GRD. Lip reconstruction. Plast Reconstr Surg 2007;120:57–64.

27. Sadove RC, Luce EA, McGrath PC. Reconstruction of the lower lip and chin with the composite radial forearm-palmaris longus free flap. Plast Reconstr Surg 1991;88:209–14.

28. Krunic AL, Weitzul S, Taylor RS. Advanced reconstructive techniques for the lip and perioral area. Dermatol Clin 2005;23:43–53.

29. Eguchi T, Nakatsuka T, Mori Y, et al. Total reconstruction of the upper lip after resection of a malignant melanoma. Scand J Plast Reconstr Surg Hand Surg 2005;39:45–7.

30. Borsuk ED, Christensen J, Dorafshar AH, et al. Aesthetic microvascular periorbital subunit reconstruction: beyond primary repair. Plast Reconstr Surg 2013;131:337–47.

31. Irish J, Gullane PJ, Gentili F, et al. Tumors of the skull base: outcome and survival analysis of 77 cases. Head Neck 1994;16:3–10.

32. Mah E, Novak CB, Zhong T, et al. Skull base reconstruction. In: Boyd BJ, Jones N, editors. Operative Microsurgery. Chapter 34. New York: McGraw Hill Education; 2015. p. 399–406.

33. Ross G, Yla-Kotola TM, Goldstein D, et al. Second free flaps in head and neck reconstruction. J Plast Reconstr Aesthet Surg 2012;65:1165–8.

Management of Unfavorable Outcomes in Head and Neck Free Flap Reconstruction

Experience-Based Lessons from the MD Anderson Cancer Center

Edward I. Chang, MD, Matthew M. Hanasono, MD,
Charles E. Butler, MD*

KEYWORDS

- Surgical flaps • Complications • Microsurgery • Thrombosis • Head and neck free flap
- Free flap loss

KEY POINTS

- Microvascular head and neck reconstruction aims to restore form and function and poses unique challenges for the reconstructive surgeon, and complications can be devastating.
- Maximizing success in free flap head and neck reconstruction requires diligent preoperative planning, appropriate flap selection, and precise surgical technique and postoperative monitoring and management.
- Compromised flap perfusion mandates early detection and definitive exploration and intervention to maximize flap salvage rates.
- Complications unrelated to the microvascular anastomosis and perfusion of the flap unfortunately are inevitable; however, appropriate management requires prompt recognition and often aggressive intervention.

INTRODUCTION

Success rates in microvascular head and neck reconstruction are greater than 95% in most high-volume institutions.[1–3] However, despite these high success rates, there remains a percentage of patients who suffer the catastrophic consequence of losing a free flap or other complications even with a successful free flap, which for head and neck defects can be incompatible with life. Patients undergoing reconstruction following tumor extirpation present unique challenges to the reconstructive microsurgeon given the high prevalence of tobacco use, malnutrition, prior or postoperative radiation damage, and history of prior surgeries. However, successful reconstruction is not simply achieving high flap survival rates, but

Disclosures: The authors have no commercial associations or financial disclosures that might pose or create a conflict of interest with information presented in this article.

Funding: No external funding was received for this study.

Department of Plastic Surgery, The University of Texas MD Anderson Cancer Center, 1515 Holcombe Boulevard, Houston, TX 77030, USA

* Corresponding author. Department of Plastic Surgery, Unit 1488, 1515 Holcombe Boulevard, Houston, TX 77030.

E-mail address: cbutler@mdanderson.org

Clin Plastic Surg 43 (2016) 653–667
http://dx.doi.org/10.1016/j.cps.2016.05.001
0094-1298/16/$ – see front matter Published by Elsevier Inc.

is also aimed at optimizing form and function and minimizing nonmicrosurgical complications. These objectives require appropriate flap selection and design, careful preoperative planning and meticulous technique, and diligent postoperative monitoring with a low threshold for definitive operative exploration for any suspicion of compromised flap perfusion. Despite a successful flap and recovery, patients do still suffer from complications. This article provides a synopsis of our approach to maximizing flap success and managing unfavorable outcomes. Many other centers have otolaryngologists performing some or all of the head and neck reconstructions. The head and neck reconstruction experience at The University of Texas MD Anderson Cancer Center is unique in that the plastic surgery department is responsible for all of the high-volume (300–400 free flaps per year) reconstructions, which we hope helps reconstructive microsurgeons worldwide.

DEFECT-SPECIFIC RECONSTRUCTION

Head and neck reconstruction aims to restore form and function and particularly for extensive defects, free tissue transfer represents the best option for achieving the most optimal outcomes. The selection for donor sites largely depends on the extent and type of defect and patient body habitus and available donor sites taking into consideration surgeon comfort and experience. Over the years, we have developed our algorithmic approach to reconstruction of head and neck defects to minimize complications and optimize outcomes, which corresponds with algorithms from other high-volume institutions.[4,5]

At our institution, we favor osteocutaneous free flaps for composite defects of the maxilla or mandible; however, in certain circumstances, soft tissue flaps are used. For example, mandibular defects, with the condyle sacrificed and the defect not extending anterior to the parasymphysis, soft tissue flaps often provide adequate postoperative function.[6] This approach applies to reconstruction following oncologic resection and for cases of osteoradionecrosis (ORN).[7] Similarly for defects involving the maxilla, a soft tissue flap may be sufficient if the alveolar bone defect does not extend beyond the canine tooth; however, for more extensive defects a bony reconstruction is indicated.[8,9]

For mucosal defects of the floor of mouth or inner cheek, we prefer a thin pliable flap, which in our patient population is a forearm-based flap, but occasionally an anterolateral thigh (ALT) flap can be used in thinner patients.[10,11] A similar algorithm is used for reconstruction of glossectomy defects where a thinner more pliable flap, such as a forearm or thin perforator ALT, is used for partial or hemiglossectomy defects, whereas a bulkier flap, such as a combined ALT/vastus lateralis flap or a rectus abdominis myocutaneous (RAM) flap, may be necessary for a subtotal or total glossectomy defect.[12] Reconstruction of extensive defects, such as those involving the tongue and the mandible, may often require the use of two free flaps to restore and optimize form and function, which can be performed safely with excellent success rates and outcomes (**Fig. 1**).[13] Similarly, for through-and-through defects, two free flaps are often necessary for reconstruction of the intraoral defect and provide coverage for the external skin.[13,14]

Reconstruction of pharyngoesophageal defects results in fewer complications and superior function if a portion of the pharyngeal or esophageal wall is preserved.[15] The ALT flap represents our flap of choice for near-total and circumferential defects especially in the setting of prior radiation and surgery where a neck resurfacing may be necessary.[16,17] In such circumstances, an ALT with two independent skin islands is used to reconstruct the pharyngoesophageal defect and provide coverage of the neck (**Fig. 2**). We reserve jejunal free flaps as a second-line option for cervical esophageal defects and the supercharged jejunal conduit for total esophagectomy defects when the option of a gastric pull-up is not possible.[18] In addition to avoiding a laparotomy, our experience is that a fasciocutaneous flap provides superior speech rehabilitation compared with intestinal flaps with comparable swallowing function. In our series of 349 cases, circumferential defects not surprisingly are associated with increased complications including fistula and strictures, and therefore preservation of any viable mucosa is critical for maximizing outcomes and providing patients with a successful reconstruction.[15] Although rare, tracheal defects can also be successfully reconstructed using free tissue transfer,[19,20] and even when coupled to esophageal disease, such extensive defects can still be salvaged with the use of fasciocutaneous free flaps and supercharged jejunal flaps.[21]

Finally, scalp reconstruction is determined based on the size of the defect. Local scalp flaps and rotation flaps are generally used for small defects. Successful reconstruction of larger defects is achieved with either free muscle or fasciocutaneous flaps with equivalent outcomes. For larger defects, the latissimus dorsi muscle with a skin graft is the flap of choice. When defects also require a cranioplasty for reconstruction of the

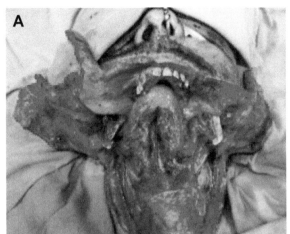

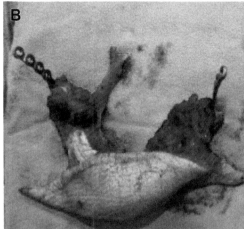

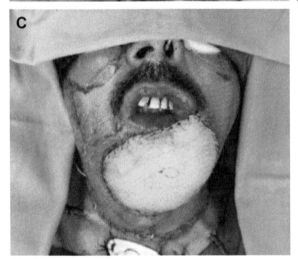

Fig. 1. (*A*) Extensive defect resulting in through-and-through composite mandibulectomy defect requiring bony reconstruction of the mandible and soft tissue coverage. (*B*) Free fibula osteocutaneous flap for reconstruction of mandible defect. (*C*) Free ALT flap for resurfacing of external skin.

calvaria, customized implants or titanium mesh have proven to be effective with low long-term complication rates.[22,23]

MANAGEMENT OF MICROVASCULAR COMPLICATIONS

Postoperative management is critical to maximizing success rates in microvascular surgery. Any concern for a microvascular complication mandates immediate evaluation by a microsurgeon with a low threshold for operative exploration.[24] Prophylactic anticoagulants, such as heparin or enoxaparin, dextran, or aspirin, have not demonstrated improved outcomes and are not routinely at our institution.[24–26] The most important factors in maximizing flap success rates are careful planning, precise technical execution, and attention to detail anticipating potential complications.[25–28] Performing an additional venous

anastomosis has not been shown to decrease complication rates or improve flap salvage and, therefore, is not recommended because a second venous outflow has been shown to decrease volumetric flow through both anastomoses.[25,29] Signs of flap compromise, such as increased swelling and bruising, change in color, and loss of the Doppler signal should prompt an immediate return to the operating room if the patient is medically stable (**Fig. 3**). Early intervention remains the single most significant predictor of flap salvage.[25–27] A negative exploration is far preferable to a lost free flap. A proposed algorithm for addressing flap compromise is summarized in **Fig. 4**.

CASE REPORTS OF UNFAVORABLE OUTCOMES
Case 1

The patient underwent a free radial forearm flap following a maxillectomy and then developed

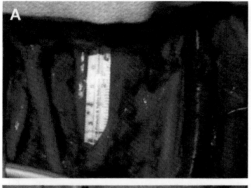

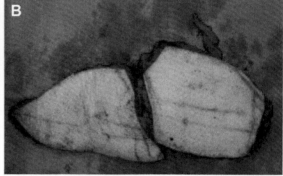

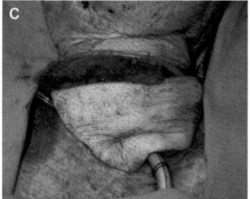

Fig. 2. (*A*) Partial pharyngectomy defect following salvage for recurrent laryngeal cancer after prior radiation. (*B*) Double skin paddle ALT for reconstruction of pharyngeal defect and (*C*) external skin resurfacing.

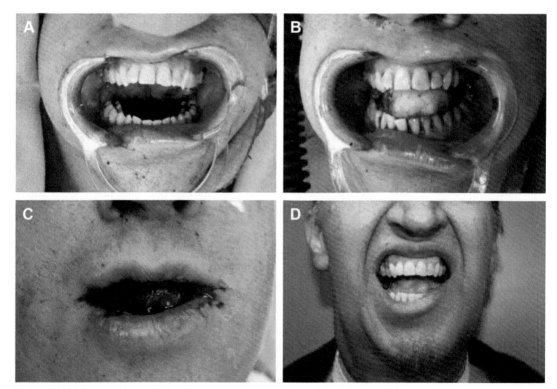

Fig. 3. (*A*) Total glossectomy defect for recurrent squamous cell carcinoma of the tongue after prior radiation therapy reconstructed with a free ALT flap (*B*). (*C*) Patient developed venous congestion of the flap on postoperative Day 1 requiring emergent exploration. (*D*) Postoperative photograph after successful flap salvage.

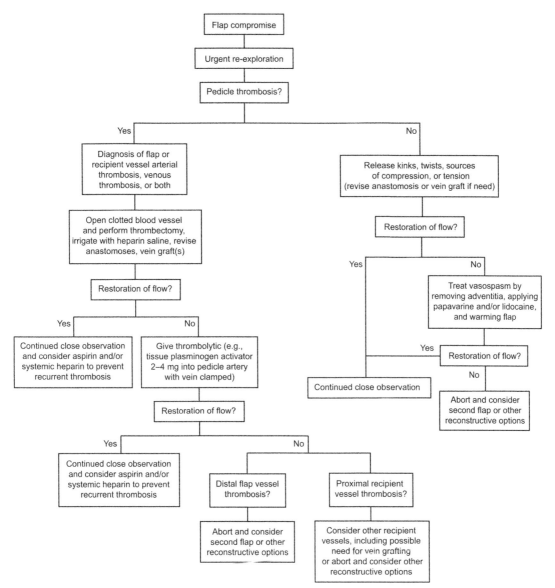

Fig. 4. MD Anderson Cancer Center plastic surgery algorithm for management of compromised free tissue transfer.

significant hollowing of the malar prominence following radiation therapy. The patient was disturbed with the cosmetic result and received two rounds of autologous fat grafting to restore the volume deficit. Although the patient achieved a reasonably aesthetic outcome, two additional operations were needed to achieve the desired result (**Fig. 5**). Given the anticipated effects of radiation, a larger flap should have been used for the initial reconstruction. A larger flap, such as an ALT or perhaps a lateral arm flap, would have provided more bulk that may have appeared excessive initially but would have settled to the appropriate size following radiation. However, alternatively, if a

larger flap were performed, there is a potential risk that the patient may need to undergo a debulking procedure if the flap is too large. Patients should be counseled regarding the need for potential revisions and autologous fat grafting or liposuction may be necessary to augment or reduce a flap to achieve the most aesthetic outcome.

Case 2

Following an extensive scalp and calvaria resection for squamous cell carcinoma, the patient had a free latissimus dorsi muscle flap for coverage with a skin graft. Unfortunately, the

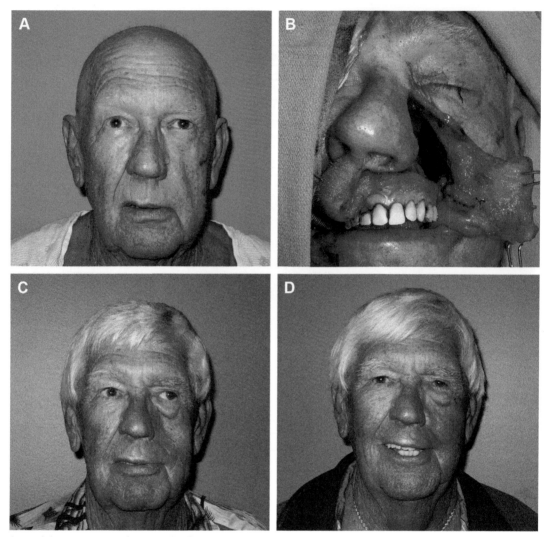

Fig. 5. (*A*) Preoperative photograph of patient before undergoing a suprastructure maxillectomy for squamous cell carcinoma (*B*) that was reconstructed with a free radial forearm flap. (*C*) Postoperative photograph after completing radiation therapy; the patient lost a noticeable amount of volume with hollowing of his malar region. (*D*) Postoperative photograph after two rounds of autologous fat grafting with improvement in the fullness of his cheek.

patient lost the distal-most aspect of the muscle requiring debridement and a second free flap to cover the exposed titanium mesh cranioplasty (**Fig. 6**). The distal portion of the latissimus dorsi muscle may not be as well perfused on the main thoracodorsal vascular pedicle and can be injured during the elevation because traction on the muscle can compromise the perfusion to the distal flap. For large defects, careful elevation of the latissimus is critical to maximize the viability of the entire flap and if the defect is too large, potentially two free flaps may be necessary. In this particular instance, likely a combination of traction on a large flap and the patient's resuming smoking led to necrosis of the distal portion. Therefore,

postoperative management and careful technique and tissue handling are equally important in avoiding unfavorable outcomes.

Case 3

The patient underwent a prior gingival resection and was found to have positive margins that ultimately required a segmental mandibulectomy that was reconstructed with a free fibula osteocutaneous free flap. The titanium plate was contoured by the dental team and used for a single segment fibula osteocutaneous flap. Postoperatively, the patient reported malocclusion with an anterior open crossbite (**Fig. 7**). The goal of

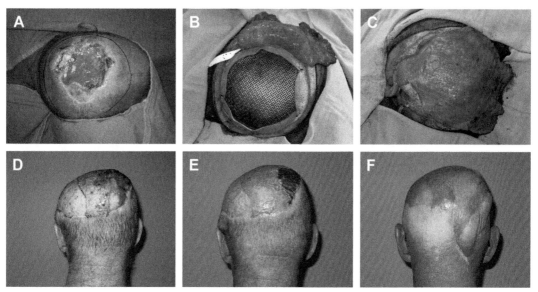

Fig. 6. (*A*) Extensive squamous cell carcinoma of the vertex of the scalp resulting in a large composite defect of the scalp soft tissue and calvaria that was reconstructed with titanium mesh (*B*) and a free latissimus dorsi muscle flap (*C*). (*D*) Postoperative photograph demonstrates loss of the distal aspect of the flap with initial loss of the skin graft and subsequently full-thickness necrosis (*E*). (*F*) Patient then underwent a second free vastus lateralis muscle flap with skin graft to cover the area of exposed titanium mesh following debridement of the necrotic latissimus flap.

mandibular reconstruction is to restore the patient's ability to eat normally and restoring class I occlusion is critical. With the increasing use of computer-assisted design and modeling, precise cutting guides are manufactured to guide the osteotomies and are coupled to titanium plates that are milled to coincide precisely with defect. Unfortunately, this technology can be prohibitively expensive. Whenever performing a fibula osteocutanous free flap for mandibular reconstruction, it is critical to contour the titanium plate yourself and to maintain the patient in class I occlusion during the fixation. Before leaving the operating room, it is important to make certain that the condyles are not dislocated from the glenoid fossa and the patient is in proper occlusion. If there is dislocation or malocclusion, it is best to correct immediately because correction of malocclusion secondarily is exceedingly challenging.

Case 4

The patient underwent a hemimaxillectomy with sacrifice of the orbital floor for adenoid cystic carcinoma. The orbital floor was reconstructed with rib graft and titanium mesh, and the maxillectomy defect was reconstructed with a free ALT flap. Following reconstruction, the patient noted diplopia that improved over time; however, he had persistent diplopia on downward gaze (**Fig. 8**). Maxillectomy defects present some of

the most challenging defects encountered by reconstructive microsurgeons especially when the orbit is involved. Maximizing outcomes should include consideration of restoring speech and swallowing, and restoring normal vision. When possible the orbital floor reconstruction should be discussed with the resecting team and ideally contouring a titanium plate should be performed before removal of the bony landmarks. The degree of soft tissue resected and intraoperative edema also present unique challenges that further complicate the microsurgeon's ability to restore the appropriate orbital volume. A forced duction test should always be performed also to ensure there is no entrapment following orbital reconstruction.

Case 5

The patient underwent a right extended orbital exenteration, including removal of the orbital floor, medial orbital wall, and a portion of the frontal sinus for a periorbital malignancy. He was reconstructed with an ALT free flap anastomosed to the superficial temporal artery and vein. He received postoperative radiation therapy. Several months later, he developed a fistula medially along the prior incision line that communicated with his nasal cavity and frontal sinus (**Fig. 9**). He returned to the operating room where the prior flap was excised and the frontal sinus was unroofed, debrided of necrotic bone, and all mucosal remnants were removed.

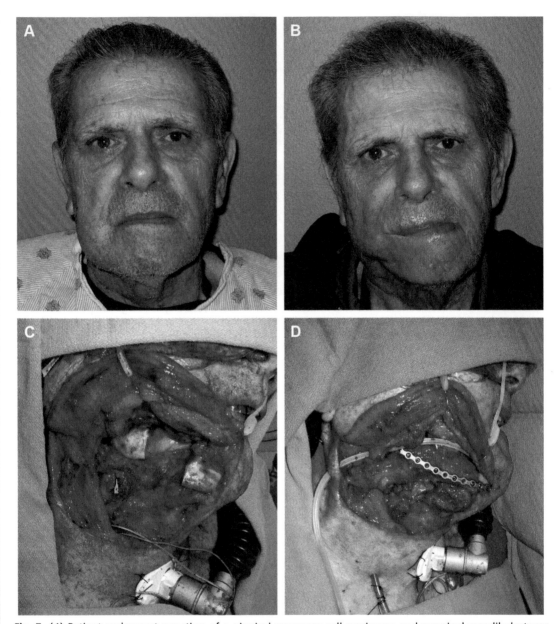

Fig. 7. (A) Patient underwent resection of a gingival squamous cell carcinoma and marginal mandibulectomy found to have more extensive disease requiring a segmentation mandibulectomy. (B) Postoperative photograph demonstrating significant malocclusion with a crossbite. (C) Segmental mandibulectomy defect and reconstruction with a free fibula osteocutaneous free flap (D).

A second ALT free flap was performed to close the defect and obliterate the frontal sinus. Such sinonasocutaneous fistulae are not uncommon following orbital exenteration and maxillectomy. Some combination of air pressure, chronic sinonasal infection, and in some cases osteoradionecrotic bone likely contribute to the development of late fistulae along the suture line between the flap and nose or between the cheek and the nose. Meticulous, multilayered closure of the wound is the key to preventing fistulae. When one does occur, it has been our experience that a second free flap that obliterates open sinuses is needed to close the defect because local options invariably result in closure of the wound over an airspace that rapidly refistulizes.

SECONDARY FREE FLAP RECONSTRUCTION

In the setting when a second free flap is planned, careful consideration should be given to placing

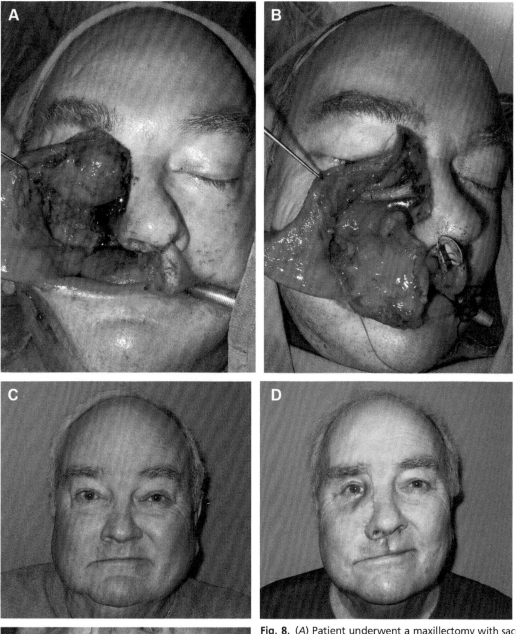

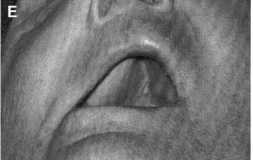

Fig. 8. (*A*) Patient underwent a maxillectomy with sacrifice of the orbital floor. (*B*) Reconstruction was performed with a free ALT flap and a rib graft with titanium mesh for the orbital floor defect. Preoperative (*C*) and postoperative (*D*) photographs of patient following reconstruction with vertical dystopia. (*E*) Intraoral skin paddle of ALT flap.

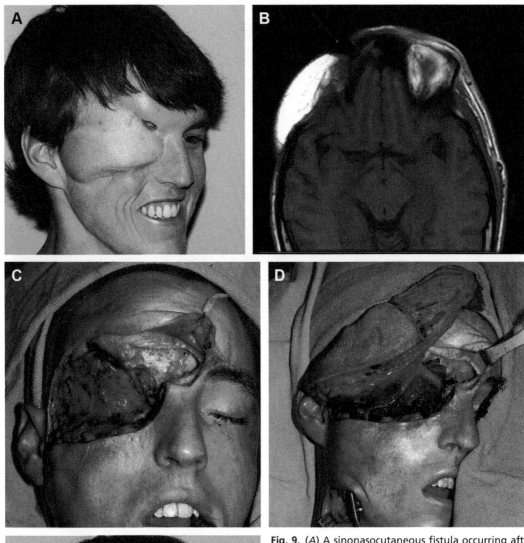

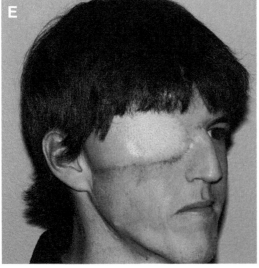

Fig. 9. (*A*) A sinonasocutaneous fistula occurring after an extended orbital exenteration reconstructed with an ALT free flap, followed by postoperative radiation therapy. (*B*) MRI demonstrating communication of the cutaneous opening with the frontal sinus. (*C*) The prior free flap was debrided and the frontal sinus was unroofed, removing all necrotic bone and providing exposure for sinus obliteration. (*D*) Inset of a second ALT free flap in which a portion of the vastus lateralis muscle was used to obliterate the maxillary sinus and a portion of the skin paddle was de-epithelialized to obliterate the frontal sinus. (*E*) The patient seen approximately 6 months after secondary reconstruction without recurrence of the fistula.

the patient through another extensive operation that is potentially subject to further complications or a flap loss.[30,31] In general, a second free flap is performed at our institution to correct complications, such as a flap loss, orocutaneous or sinonasocutaneous fistula, ORN, stricture, or to improve the cosmetic result. In certain circumstances, patients may be better reconstructed using another modality rather than a second free flap, such as local flaps or potentially even prosthesis.[32,33] However, despite the added complexity of performing a secondary free flap in a patient who has already had free flap, our experience and others have demonstrated excellent success rates.[34,35]

When a secondary free flap is performed, particularly in the setting of a prior neck dissection, radiation, and a primary free flap, other factors become increasingly important. In particular, the reconstructive microsurgeon needs to pay attention to the availability of recipient vessels and should consider an angiogram and the use of alternate recipient vessels, such as the transverse cervical vessels or the need for vein grafts.[36,37] Dissecting additional recipients in a previously radiated field following a neck dissection is fraught with high risks in the frozen neck and should be avoided.

Aside from the need for recipient vessels, soft tissue coverage of the neck can also be challenging. Given the lack of recipient vessels, a second free flap may be exceedingly challenging unless a flow-through flap is performed.[37] However, occasionally if multiple perforators exist, potentially a second skin island can be harvested and used for neck resurfacing.[38] If none of these options are available, local pedicle flaps, such as the pectoralis major muscle flap or an internal mammary artery perforator flap, can be used reliably and effectively.

MANAGEMENT OF UNFAVORABLE POSTOPERATIVE COMPLICATIONS

Aside from complications associated with the microvascular anastomosis, patients undergoing free flap reconstruction are potentially at risk for several other complications even in the setting of a successful free flap. Often, patients undergoing such extensive resections and reconstructive operations are malnourished, have had prior radiation and chemotherapy, and have had a history of or may be actively using tobacco products. Consequently, these patients are potentially at risk for delayed wound healing of the flap and the donor sites, fistula, infection, and medical complications. All patients should undergo a thorough medical evaluation to optimize patients before embarking on an extensive resection and microvascular reconstruction.

In general, many complications are managed conservatively with antibiotics for superficial infections, and local wound care and dressing changes for wound dehiscence. However, cellulitis in the neck that does not resolve with intravenous antibiotics may suggest an abscess or fistula. A computed tomography scan may be useful in identifying and localizing an abscess, seroma, or a leak. In general, we have a low threshold for operative intervention if there is a suspicion for a fluid collection that can progress to an abscess or a fistula. Early, aggressive drainage and washout of a neck abscess is critical to minimize the risk of a carotid blowout. In the setting of a superficial dehiscence, local wound care may be adequate; however, if vital structures are exposed, definitive soft tissue coverage is necessary. The pectoralis major muscle or myocutaneous flap is our flap of choice for coverage and neck resurfacing in these circumstances.

However, in the setting of prior radiation and surgery, preemptive replacement of damaged neck skin with external flap coverage should be considered. Designing a flap with two independent skin paddles based on individual perforators for reconstruction of the primary defect and the neck obviates suturing radiated tissue together and may minimize the risk of wound dehiscence.[11,36] In certain circumstances, a second free flap or a pedicle pectoralis muscle flap with a skin graft is used for neck coverage; however, consideration should be given to the increased operative time and donor site morbidity when a single free flap may have sufficed.

MANAGEMENT OF FISTULA

Free flap reconstruction of complex head and neck defects is fraught with risks and unique complications, such as a fistula, which can potentially lead to flap failure or death if a patient suffers a carotid blowout. A low index of suspicion should predominate all patients who have received preoperative radiation, chemotherapy, and surgery. Prolonged swelling, increasing erythema, malodorous or purulent discharge, or changes in drain output should all prompt further evaluation. Patients may or may not exhibit leukocytosis and fever. A computed tomography scan or barium swallow may be indicated to evaluate for the possibility of the fistula but are not required for an obvious fistula. A so-called "herald bleed" represents a potential emergency that warrants urgent exploration to avoid a life-threatening complication. We generally manage fistula with one or more operative or bedside irrigation and debridement procedures until the wound is clean before performing definitive repair, usually with a pectoralis major muscle or myocutaneous flap. Culture-directed antibiotic treatment is also indicated. Performing a free flap in a grossly infected field is associated with an elevated risk of failure and is not recommended.

MANAGEMENT OF STRICTURES

Patients undergoing reconstruction of pharyngoesophageal defects should also be counseled on the risks of developing a stricture that can have a dramatic impact on patients' function and quality of life. We have previously demonstrated that circumferential defects are at increased risk for stricture formation, and therefore preservation of a posterior strip of mucosa affords some advantage for swallowing function following reconstruction.[15] However, in certain circumstances it is not possible to avoid a circumferential resection, and in these cases, it is important to interrupt the circumferential scar at the distal anastomosis. We typically recommend designing the flap with a "dart" that is inset into a longitudinal myotomy in the cervical esophagus to increase the functional circumference of the anastomosis. Not only does this aid in widening the functional diameter of the distal anastomosis, but it also interrupts a circular scar that is more prone to stricture formation. Despite these efforts, patients can still suffer from a cicatricial stricture, which is relieved by serial dilations. In the rare setting of severe strictures recalcitrant to dilation, operative intervention with a second flap may be necessary. In certain circumstances, dysphagia may actually represent recurrent disease. In these circumstances, a secondary operation for resection may be indicated and performing a second free flap has been found to achieve equivalent success rates with excellent postoperative speaking and swallowing function.[35]

MANAGEMENT OF OSTEORADIONECROSIS

Treatment of head and neck malignancies often requires radiation therapy, which presents significant challenges to the reconstructive microsurgeon. ORN is a complication that can result following radiation treatment and often is more difficult to reconstruct than a primary defect following tumor extirpation. Patients may present with significant trismus, pain, recurrent infection, an orocutaneous fistula, or a pathologic fracture. In some situations, patients may present with

ORN following adjuvant radiation for treatment of a head and neck malignancy when a free flap has already been performed. This increases the complexity of the reconstruction given the prior scarring from surgery, need for additional recipient vessels, and significant radiation damage. The previously radiated and operated neck presents unique challenges that need to be considered because the anatomy is often distorted and the natural tissue planes are lost. Similarly, isolation of recipient vessels in the field can also be risky and dangerous. Consideration should be given to using alternate recipient vessels, and vein grafts may be necessary and should also be considered when treating patients for ORN. Furthermore, special consideration should also be given to resurfacing of the neck as previously discussed. This may require modification of flap design and the need for multiple perforators, or it may require a second free flap or a pedicle pectoralis major flap for neck coverage (**Fig. 10**).

In general, we recommend proceeding with free flap reconstruction for symptomatic ORN defects, which affords superior postoperative function for most patients. Although osteocutaneous flaps were associated with increased complications compared with soft tissue flaps, bony reconstruction can still be performed safely with low complication and flap loss rates.[7] Patients undergoing bony reconstruction for ORN are candidates for dental rehabilitation with dental implants, which provides significant improvements to patients' overall quality of life following reconstruction, because irradiated, necrotic bone is being replaced with healthy, well-vascularized bone.[39]

DONOR SITE COMPLICATIONS

Prospective studies regarding donor site morbidity of the more common free flaps performed at our institution have demonstrated acceptable low risk of complications with the ALT flap and the free fibula osteocutaneous free flap.[40,41] In general, most infections, wound dehiscence, and superficial complications are avoided with careful tissue handling, meticulous technique, tension-free closure, and appropriate care of skin grafts. Despite the high percentage (84%) of patients who reported numbness in the distribution of the lateral femoral cutaneous nerve distribution after undergoing ALT flap, all patients nonetheless regained their preoperative functional status without permanent debilitation or sequelae after recovering from the operation.[40]

Analysis of 127 consecutive patients undergoing a free fibula flap demonstrated approximately a third of patients suffered a complication in the

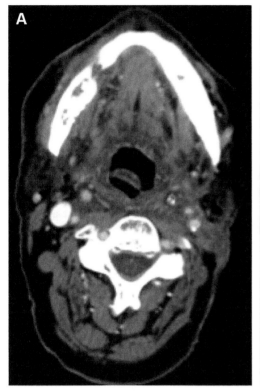

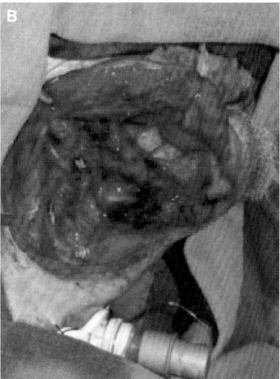

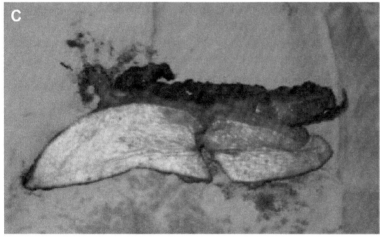

Fig. 10. (*A*) Patient with osteoradionecrosis who presented with a pathologic fracture and trismus following radiation treatment of tonsillar squamous cell carcinoma underwent composite resection with needle for skin resurfacing (*B*). (*C*) A double skin paddle free fibula flap was performed to reconstruct the intraoral defect and provide coverage of the external skin.

perioperative period, including skin graft loss (15%), infection (11%), and wound dehiscence (8%). Furthermore, 8% reported weakness, 9% noted flexion disturbance of the great toe, 12% reported reduced ankle mobility, and 4% complained of decreased ankle stability. Nonetheless, 96% of patients returned back to their baseline, preoperative functional status following reconstruction.[41]

Harvest of a forearm flap often requires a skin graft to resurface the donor site, which may be at risk for partial loss and exposure of the tendons. An ulnar artery perforator flap reportedly has lower risks of tendon exposure because the donor site typically overlies the muscle of the ulnar forearm.[10] Regardless, local wound care is often sufficient in treating minor wound complications. Other reported complications, such as cold intolerance, decreased strength, and diminished sensation, should also be discussed with patients; however, these typically have not caused significant complications in our patients. In general, a suprafascial harvest of forearm flaps preserves an additional layer of fascia over the tendons and can improve skin graft take, thereby reducing the risks of poor skin graft take to the forearm donor site.[10,42]

In the setting of large extensive head and neck defects, an abdominal flap may be necessary, such as a vertical RAM flap or transverse RAM flap.[43] Harvest of an abdominal flap should proceed in a muscle-sparing and fascia-preserving fashion similar to harvesting of an abdominal flap for breast reconstruction to minimize donor site morbidity.[44] In the setting that a significant amount of fascia is sacrificed, the use of a component separation or reinforcement with mesh has proven to significantly reduce postoperative bulge and hernia rates.[44,45]

DISCUSSION

Microvascular free flap head and neck reconstruction has witnessed tremendous advances over the years and success rates have improved significantly. Maximizing success rates depends on several factors including careful flap design and selection, appropriate recipient vessel selection and surgical technique, and diligent postoperative management. However, even in the setting of a successful free flap, a second free flap may still be necessary to correct complications, such as fistulae, stricture, ORN, or to improve the cosmetic result. Optimizing outcomes for patients may require revision surgery with debulking or fat grafting to improve the overall cosmetic result. Functional complications, such as malocclusion, diplopia, and partial flap necrosis, present significant complications that are much more challenging to correct and often are avoided with careful planning and attention to details.

SUMMARY

Free flap head and neck reconstruction is performed safely and reliably with high success rates. However, optimizing outcomes and maximizing success rates is multifactorial. Careful preoperative management and flap design, meticulous flap dissection and surgical technique, diligent postoperative monitoring, and aggressive operative intervention in the setting of complications are critical in achieving the objectives of a successful reconstruction and restoring form and function for patients undergoing treatment of head and neck cancers.

REFERENCES

1. Bui DT, Cordeiro PG, Hu QY, et al. Free flap reexploration: indications, treatment, and outcomes in 1193 free flaps. Plast Reconstr Surg 2007; 119(7):2092–100.
2. Mirzabeigi MN, Wang T, Kovach SJ, et al. Free flap take-back following postoperative microvascular compromise: predicting salvage versus failure. Plast Reconstr Surg 2012;130(3):579–89.
3. Cannady SB, Rosenthal EL, Knott PD, et al. Free tissue transfer for head and neck reconstruction: a contemporary review. JAMA Facial Plast Surg 2014;16(5):367–73.
4. Wong CH, Wei FC. Microsurgical free flap in head and neck reconstruction. Head Neck 2010;32(9): 1236–45.
5. Chim H, Salgado CJ, Seselgyte R, et al. Principles of head and neck reconstruction: an algorithm to guide flap selection. Semin Plast Surg 2010;24(2): 148–54.
6. Hanasono MM, Zevallos JP, Skoracki RJ, et al. A prospective analysis of bony versus soft-tissue reconstruction for posterior mandibular defects. Plast Reconstr Surg 2010;125(5):1413–21.
7. Baumann DP, Yu P, Hanasono MM, et al. Free flap reconstruction of osteoradionecrosis of the mandible: a 10-year review and defect classification. Head Neck 2011;33(6):800–7.
8. Hanasono MM, Silva AK, Yu P, et al. A comprehensive algorithm for oncologic maxillary reconstruction. Plast Reconstr Surg 2013;131(1): 47–60.
9. Hanasono MM, Skoracki RJ. The omega-shaped fibula osteocutaneous free flap for reconstruction of extensive midfacial defects. Plast Reconstr Surg 2010;125(4):160e–2e.
10. Yu P, Chang EI, Selber JC, et al. Perforator patterns of the ulnar artery perforator flap. Plast Reconstr Surg 2012;129(1):213–20.
11. Lin SJ, Rabie A, Yu P. Designing the anterolateral thigh flap without preoperative Doppler or imaging. J Reconstr Microsurg 2010;26(1):67–72.
12. Chang EI, Yu P, Skoracki RJ, et al. Comprehensive analysis of functional outcomes and survival after microvascular reconstruction of glossectomy defects. Ann Surg Oncol 2015;22(9):3061–9.
13. Hanasono MM, Weinstock YE, Yu P. Reconstruction of extensive head and neck defects with multiple simultaneous free flaps. Plast Reconstr Surg 2008; 122(6):1739–46.
14. Wei FC, Yazar S, Lin CH, et al. Double free flaps in head and neck reconstruction. Clin Plast Surg 2005;32(3):303–8.
15. Selber JC, Xue A, Liu J, et al. Pharyngoesophageal reconstruction outcomes following 349 cases. J Reconstr Microsurg 2014;30(9):641–54.
16. Yu P, Hanasono MM, Skoracki RJ, et al. Pharyngoesophageal reconstruction with the anterolateral thigh flap after total laryngopharyngectomy. Cancer 2010; 116(7):1718–24.

17. Yu P, Lewin JS, Reece GP, et al. Comparison of clinical and functional outcomes and hospital costs following pharyngoesophageal reconstruction with the anterolateral thigh free flap versus the jejunal flap. Plast Reconstr Surg 2006;117(3):968–74.

18. Poh M, Selber JC, Skoracki R, et al. Technical challenges of total esophageal reconstruction using a supercharged jejunal flap. Ann Surg 2011;253(6): 1122–9.

19. Yu P, Clayman GL, Walsh GL. Long-term outcomes of microsurgical reconstruction for large tracheal defects. Cancer 2011;117(4):802–8.

20. Yu P, Clayman GL, Walsh GL. Human tracheal reconstruction with a composite radial forearm free flap and prosthesis. Ann Thorac Surg 2006;81(2): 714–6.

21. Ghali S, Chang EI, Rice DC, et al. Microsurgical reconstruction of combined tracheal and total esophageal defects. J Thorac Cardiovasc Surg 2015;150(5):1261–6.

22. Lee EI, Chao AH, Skoracki RJ, et al. Outcomes of calvarial reconstruction in cancer patients. Plast Reconstr Surg 2014;133(3):675–82.

23. Chao AH, Yu P, Skoracki RJ, et al. Microsurgical reconstruction of composite scalp and calvarial defects in patients with cancer: a 10-year experience. Head Neck 2012;34(12):1759–64.

24. Hanasono MM, Butler CE. Prevention and treatment of thrombosis in microvascular surgery. J Reconstr Microsurg 2008;24(5):305–14.

25. Chang EI, Zhang H, Liu J, et al. Analysis of risk factors for flap loss and salvage in free flap head and neck reconstruction. Head Neck 2016;38(Suppl 1): E771–5.

26. Chen KT, Mardini S, Chuang DC, et al. Timing of presentation of the first signs of vascular compromise dictates the salvage outcome of free flap transfers. Plast Reconstr Surg 2007;120(1):187–95.

27. Yu P, Chang DW, Miller MJ, et al. Analysis of 49 cases of flap compromise in 1310 free flaps for head and neck reconstruction. Head Neck 2009; 31(1):45–51.

28. Chang EI. My first 100 consecutive microvascular free flaps: pearls and lessons learned in first year of practice. Plast Reconstr Surg Glob Open 2013; 1(4):e27.

29. Hanasono MM, Kocak E, Ogunleye O, et al. One versus two venous anastomoses in microvascular free flap surgery. Plast Reconstr Surg 2010;126(5): 1548–57.

30. Selber JC, Angel Soto-Miranda M, Liu J, et al. The survival curve: factors impacting the outcome of free flap take-backs. Plast Reconstr Surg 2012; 130(1):105–13.

31. Corbitt C, Skoracki RJ, Yu P, et al. Free flap failure in head and neck reconstruction. Head Neck 2014; 36(10):1440–5.

32. Kim JY, Buck DW 2nd, Johnson SA, et al. The temporoparietal fascial flap is an alternative to free flaps for orbitomaxillary reconstruction. Plast Reconstr Surg 2010;126(3):880–8.

33. Moreno MA, Skoracki RJ, Hanna EY, et al. Microvascular free flap reconstruction versus palatal obturation for maxillectomy defects. Head Neck 2010; 32(7):860–8.

34. Wei FC, Demirkan F, Chen HC, et al. The outcome of failed free flap in head and neck and extremity reconstruction: what is next in the reconstructive ladder? Plast Reconstr Surg 2001; 108:1154–60.

35. Hanasono MM, Corbitt CA, Yu P, et al. Success of sequential free flaps in head and neck reconstruction. J Plast Reconstr Aesthet Surg 2014;67(9): 1186–93.

36. Yu P. The transverse cervical vessels as recipient vessels for previously treated head and neck cancer patients. Plast Reconstr Surg 2005;115(5): 1253–8.

37. Hanasono MM, Barnea Y, Skoracki RJ. Microvascular surgery in the previously operated and irradiated neck. Microsurgery 2009;29(1):1–7.

38. Yu P, Chang EI, Hanasono MM. Design of a reliable skin paddle for the fibula osteocutaneous flap: perforator anatomy revisited. Plast Reconstr Surg 2011;128(2):440–6.

39. Ch'ng S, Skoracki RJ, Selber JC, et al. Osseointegrated implant based dental rehabilitation in head and neck reconstruction patients. Head Neck 2016;38(Suppl 1):E321–7.

40. Hanasono MM, Skoracki RJ, Yu P. A prospective study of donor-site morbidity after anterolateral thigh fasciocutaneous and myocutaneous free flap harvest in 220 patients. Plast Reconstr Surg 2010; 125(1):209–14.

41. Momoh AO, Yu P, Skoracki RJ, et al. A prospective cohort study of fibula free flap donor-site morbidity in 157 consecutive patients. Plast Reconstr Surg 2011;128(3):714–20.

42. Wong CH, Lin JY, Wei FC. The bottom-up approach to the suprafascial harvest of the radial forearm flap. Am J Surg 2008;196(5):e60–4.

43. Butler CE, Lewin JS. Reconstruction of large composite oromandibulomaxillary defects with free vertical rectus abdominis myocutaneous flaps. Plast Reconstr Surg 2004;113(2):499–507.

44. Chang EI, Chang EI, Soto-Miranda MA, et al. Comprehensive analysis of donor-site morbidity in abdominally based free flap breast reconstruction. Plast Reconstr Surg 2013;132(6): 1383–91.

45. Baumann DP, Butler CE. Component separation improves outcomes in VRAM flap donor sites with excessive fascial tension. Plast Reconstr Surg 2010;126(5):1573–80.

Mayo Clinic Experience with Unfavorable Results After Free Tissue Transfer to Head and Neck

Thomas H. Nagel, MD, Richard E. Hayden, MD*

KEYWORDS

• Head and neck reconstruction • Microsurgery • Free flap • Salvage

KEY POINTS

• Successful free tissue transfer should produce optimal functional as well as aesthetic outcomes. Anticipating potential risk factors before reconstruction is key.
• Specific factors negatively affecting head and neck reconstruction include radiation, contamination, and mobility. Of these, radiation with its attendant damage to the capillary bed provides the biggest challenge.
• Poor wound healing due to these factors can lead to wound breakdown and fistula formation, threatening the microvascular anastomoses, the flap, and the great vessels of the neck.
• Maxillo-mandibular reconstruction must respect the occlusal plane for functional dental rehabilitation to be optimized.
• Reconstruction of the pharynx and esophagus following chemoradiotherapy must factor in the ongoing negative effects that can obliterate laryngo-pharyngo-esophageal function.

INTRODUCTION

The aim of this article is to share our experience with head and neck reconstructive surgery and technical approaches we have learned from untoward results. There are several factors somewhat unique to the head and neck patient population that challenge the reconstructive surgeon.

First, the upper aerodigestive tract contaminates the reconstructed area. Second, mobility of reconstructed tissue is to be expected and can impact healing. Third, radiotherapy (RT) in the upper aerodigestive tract either before or after reconstructive surgery is the norm. The negative tissue side effects created by radiation need to be factored into the technical considerations of

each surgery. Most of the discussion regarding RT references patients who have already undergone radiation because a deficient vascular bed presents unique challenges to healing. Current use of concurrent chemoradiotherapy (CXRT) produces even greater tissue damage than conventional RT.

The last and perhaps one of the most important aspects of head and neck reconstruction relates to how patients meet their world. Appearance that includes functional and aesthetic outcomes is equally or more important following head and neck reconstruction than anywhere else in the body. As we set expectations for our patients, we outline tiers of priority: oncologic success,

Disclosure Statement: The authors have nothing to disclose.
Department of Otolaryngology-Head and Neck Surgery, Mayo Clinic, 5777 East Mayo Boulevard, Phoenix, AZ 85054, USA
* Corresponding author.
E-mail address: hayden.richard@mayo.edu

Clin Plastic Surg 43 (2016) 669–682
http://dx.doi.org/10.1016/j.cps.2016.05.005

function, and appearance. Although these goals must be prioritized in this order, the importance of function, namely, speech and swallowing, and appearance are essential to successful head and neck reconstruction and cannot be overemphasized.

SALVAGING FREE FLAPS

Modern reconstructive surgeons can expect a better than 98% success rate with free tissue transfer.[1–3] Improvements in microsurgical training, surgical instruments, and technique; the expansion of potential free tissue donor sites; and a better understanding of free tissue physiology have certainly contributed to the current high rates of success.

As we reviewed our experience of more than 2500 flaps, exclusively in the head and neck, we have seen our failure rates in the last 2 decades plateau at less than 1%. There remain 2% to 3% of cases that have early vascular compromise and require salvage. Most cases of vascular compromise are venous pedicle obstructions, and most of these occur within 72 hours after surgery. A very small number of arterial pedicle problems are discussed later. Our practice is not unique in that careful postoperative monitoring is used for early identification of flap compromise with urgent return to the operating room (OR) when necessary and leech therapy for temporary venous decongestion of the flap while preparing for the OR.

Our protocol for dealing with venous thrombosis is based on lessons learned from untoward results. Failure to trim microstay sutures following anastomosis can result in inadvertent traction on the microvascular anastomoses during even the most gentle clot removal in those patients with hematomas in the neck surrounding the anastomoses. Our technique has not fundamentally changed for 30 years. When all blood clots have been completely removed in the neck and an engorged venous pedicle is identified together with a patent arterial pedicle, the venous pedicle is sectioned at the anastomosis. A mechanical thrombectomy of the venous pedicle is performed, which by itself rarely, if ever, restores flow. The recipient artery is clamped proximal to the arterial anastomosis, and intra-arterial injection of a thrombolytic is administered. This practice has changed over 30 years from streptokinase to urokinase to the tissue plasminogen activator (TPA) currently used. The concentration of thrombolytic can be much greater than a systemic dose as the agent will not enter the systemic circulation because the venous pedicle has been severed. The arterial clamp is removed, and the agent can work its way into the

flap. Retrograde irrigation with the same high concentration of thrombolytic is performed. Sometimes with engorged thrombosed veins within the venous system of the flap, intravenous injections of these veins are also performed with the concentrated thrombolytic. Venous outflow slowly returns, during which time all venous outflow is extracorporeal. While awaiting the return of adequate venous outflow, an alternative recipient vein is prepared. Depending on the patient, this may be the original shortened vein, a new vein, or even a vein graft in exceptional cases. Once full venous outflow has been reestablished and all injected thrombolytic has been flushed from the flap, the venous anastomosis is performed (**Fig. 1**). We do not routinely anticoagulate our free flap patients with anything more than aspirin or ketorolac tromethamine (Toradol). However, in salvage patients, we heparinize the patients for a few days. In the 1980s, we salvaged a dozen or more flaps using this technique and always heparinized the patients following salvage. When we decided to not heparinize one salvaged patient, rethrombosis occurred. Regardless of whether a lesson was learned from untoward results or we responded to an anecdotal experience, we now heparinize our patients after salvaging their flaps.

RADIOTHERAPY CONSIDERATIONS

The negative impact of RT and CXRT presents the greatest challenge to successful head and neck reconstructive surgery. Radiation produces subintimal fibrosis in the microvasculature of the radiated field and can dramatically decrease or even obliterate the capillary bed. This loss of the capillary bed dramatically decreases the affected tissues' nutrient and oxygen delivery system resulting in predictably compromised healing. Reconstruction in an irradiated bed will have higher rates of orocutaneous or pharyngocutaneous fistulae even when well-vascularized flaps are used. The nonradiated free flap will not heal as well to heavily radiated, poorly vascularized, contaminated, and mobile tissues. Several strategies are used to minimize the risk fistula poses to a free flap. When possible we try to locate the microvascular anastomosis to the contralateral neck, which is far less likely to become contaminated by a fistula. If a fistula seems imminent or does develop, the drainage must be redirected not only away from the carotid artery but also away from the microvascular anastomosis.

If the microvascular anastomosis must be in the ipsilateral neck, it is beneficial to devise ways to ensure that if a patient were to fistulize, the vascular anastomosis would be protected from

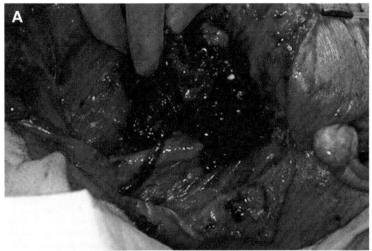

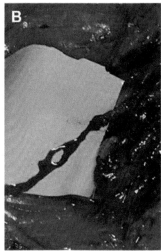

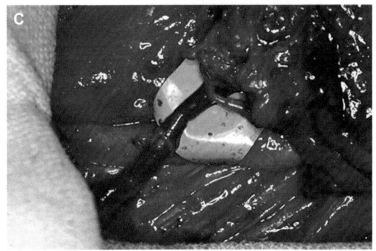

Fig. 1. Salvage of gastro-omental free flap. (*A*) Intraoperative view left neck, demonstrating complete thrombosis of the gastroepiploic vein anastomosed to the external jugular vein. (*B*) Intraoperative view after mechanical thrombectomy and TPA thrombolysis, demonstrating return of good venous outflow from the gastroepiploic vein. (*C*) Intraoperative view following successful salvage with reanastomosis of the gastroepiploic vein with shortened external jugular vein.

the drainage. One technique is to imbricate a strip of the intraoral skin paddle under intraoral suture lines. This de-epithelized imbricated skin paddle serves to shield the microanastomosis if a fistula were to develop and provides a second line of healing if intraoral suture lines were to dehisce, often avoiding a fistula. The de-epithelialized lateral aspect of the skin paddle can also be draped over the microanastomoses in the upper neck such that, if a fistula were to occur the drainage would be superficial to the paddle and thereby not affect the anastomosis.

Nonpliable radiated soft tissues also pose a problem. In cases of severe soft tissue radiation damage and a woody neck resecting more of this tissue may actually be preferred and result in fewer healing complications (**Fig. 2**). This point is particularly important if poor wound healing might result in carotid or vascular pedicle exposure. Here again, it is wise to imbricate in these cases. By

harvesting a larger flap or skin paddle than is needed, a de-epithelialized rind of the skin paddle can be imbricated beyond the suture lines with the neck skin. Then if suture lines were to separate there is still a good chance of wound healing by secondary intention without the patient suffering a full wound dehiscence.

Another byproduct of head and neck RT is osteoradionecrosis (ORN) of the mandible. During mandibulectomy for ORN it is important to ensure that the mandible resection is extended into well-vascularized, bleeding bone. Otherwise a valuable flap can be expended only to have the adjacent bone develop radionecrosis and require replacement.

In heavily radiated cases

- When possible, perform the microvascular anastomosis in the neck contralateral to a potential fistula.

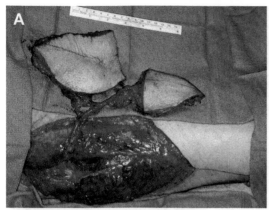
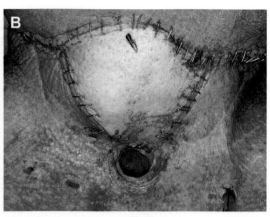
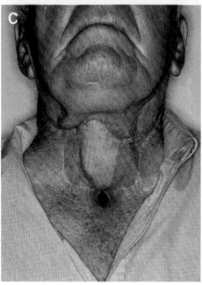

Fig. 2. Reconstruction of defect following salvage laryngophar-yngectomy and removal of poorly vascularized neck skin after failed chemoradiotherapy. (*A*) Intraoperative view demonstrating a 2-paddle anterolateral thigh flap. The larger paddle will be used to reconstruct the laryngopharyngectomy defect. The smaller paddle on the right will reconstruct the missing anterior neck skin and protect the great vessels of the neck. (*B*) Early postoperative view of the anterior neck skin replacement. (*C*) Postoperative view, 3 years later.

- Remove and replace anterior neck skin that, if compromised, would expose the micro-anastomosis, great vessels, or the flap reconstruction.
- Imbricate excess de-epithelialized flap skin under recipient tissue to minimize the conse-quences of suture line dehiscence.
- Resect the osteoradionecrotic bone back to a healthy bleeding bone.

MICROVASCULAR ARTERIAL PEDICLE RUPTURE

Radiation damage associated with ORN is not always limited to bone. We have observed that ORN serves as an indicator of the severity of the radiation damage to surrounding tissue. Radiation damages the vasa vasorum and vasa vasorae of all vessels in the radiated field, with resultant decreased flow and frequent occlu-sion.[4] Obliteration of the nutrient vessels to the arterial wall over time increases the risk of rupture.[5]

We have had a small number of recipient artery ruptures in our ORN population undergoing fibula free flap reconstruction.[6] Interestingly, these rup-tures always occurred in the recipient artery well proximal to the anastomotic suture line where the adjacent vessel wall had been subjected to adven-titial trimming and clamping. None of these cases had had fistulae or contamination around these ruptures. We postulate that mechanical and in-flammatory stress from dissecting and isolating these radiated arteries from their radiated and scarred surroundings combined with relative devascularization of their vessel walls secondary to radiation led to pseudoaneurysm and eventual rupture. Pathologic analysis of the ruptured arterial segments supports this hypothesis, demon-strating acute arteritis and pseudoaneurysm.

The time to arterial rupture ranged from 7 to 17 days. In these cases, after the anastomosis was reestablished, repeat rupture usually occurred within a week and should be anticipated. Ultimately all of these anastomoses required ligation. Despite this, we were able to salvage all of these flaps without any partial or total flap loss because flap vascularization was sustained for more than 15 days. Although delayed when compared with nonradiated native tissues, the radiated recipient surgical bed can obviously still ultimately provide neovascularization that supports the free flap restoring tissue perfusion independent of the vascular pedicle.

A real exception to this expectation is found when using jejunal or gastro-omental flaps in radiated recipient beds. Expect poor neovascularization across the serosa of these transplants.

- ORN may be an indicator of the severity of radiation injury to surrounding soft tissue.
- Mechanical and inflammatory stress accompanying harvest and preparation of recipient vessels with compromised vasa vasorum(ae) may predispose these arteries to rupture, so vessel isolation and prep should be minimized.
- If arterial rupture occurs, we think it is beneficial to revise the anastomoses with proximal artery or a new recipient artery to extend the time of flap tissue vascularization. Although one should be prepared for the high likelihood of rerupture, this may afford enough time for neovascularization from the surgical bed to support the free flap without loss even for composite flaps.

THE VESSEL-DEPLETED NECK

Previously operated and radiated (especially chemoradiated) necks may simply have no veins available for anastomosis of a free tissue transfer. This deficit is not unique to radiated necks but is far more common in tertiary/quaternary care patients who usually have already had repeat multimodality therapies on arrival. To overcome a vessel-depleted neck, one must either bring recipient vessels to the neck or use flaps with long pedicles that can reach unconventional recipient vessels below the clavicle.

Vein grafts can extend deficient vascular pedicles but bring added risks with dual anastomoses required, and we use them only as a last resort. Because of the proximity of the cephalic vein to the neck, it is a very useful option for venous outflow from the head and neck. The distal cephalic vein is sectioned in the arm and through retrograde dissection delivered to the neck with all of its branches having been secured in the arm. When anastomosed to the flap donor vein in the head and neck, the venous outflow travels anterograde through the cephalic vein to the subclavian vein (**Fig. 3**).

Some cases dictate that free tissue transfer be abandoned in favor of transferring regional tissue with its own vascular supply. The pectoralis major, trapezius, and latissimus dorsi flaps can still be important regional flaps in head and neck reconstruction. Their vascular pedicles are outside the zone of neck surgery, and the tissue components of the flaps are outside the zone of radiation. Sometimes, in patients who have had multiple operations before arrival, including one or more of these regional pedicled flaps, we have had to reanastomose the donor vessels of our free flap to the pedicle vessels of an existing pedicled flap already in the neck.

We often use the latissimus dorsi pedicled flap in necks that require a last-resort reconstructive

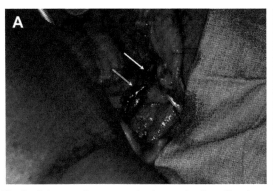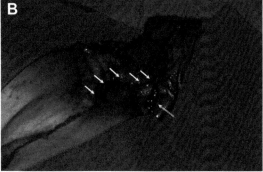

Fig. 3. Salvage of compromised scapular free flap in vessel-depleted neck. (*A*) Intraoperative view of left neck, demonstrating completely thrombosed subscapular vein (*solid arrow*) and external jugular vein (*double arrow*). Note the internal jugular vein was resected during the cancer surgery. Incision in deltoid groove to left arm to procure cephalic vein. (*B*) Intraoperative view of the left neck following successful flap salvage. The cephalic vein (*solid arrow*) has been harvested from the left upper arm and anastomosed to the subscapular vein. The thrombosed external jugular vein (*double arrow*) is seen posterior to the new venous pedicle.

tool. The latissimus flap offers much soft tissue, and the pedicle can accommodate a wide arc of rotation for delivery. A properly planned latissimus dorsi pedicle flap can reach the vertex scalp or contralateral mandible. We prefer to create a transaxillary tunnel between the pectoralis major and minor muscles, delivering the flap to the neck through a skin incision made above the clavicle. Several technical considerations have been outlined by the senior author following tunneling to prevent torsion or traction on the vascular pedicle.[7] The circumflex scapular artery should be preserved to ensure a gentle curve to the vascular pedicle, and the humeral tendon needs to be secured to adjacent rib periosteum to protect against torsion or traction on this vascular pedicle.

- Overcoming a vessel-depleted neck may require vein grafts, which add risk. The cephalic vein transferred to the neck can be a good option for venous outflow.
- In some heavily treated necks, it may be prudent to avoid free tissue transfer. Consider regionally pedicled flaps in these difficult cases.
- Remember that the vascular pedicle to a previously used pedicled flap can provide potential recipient vessels for a free flap.

RECONSTRUCTIVE CHALLENGES

Three great challenges to the head and neck reconstructive surgeon 30 years ago were (1) reconstruction of the anterior mandibular arch, (2) reconstruction of the total laryngopharyngectomy defect, and (3) reconstruction of the total glossectomy defect without laryngectomy.

RECONSTRUCTION OF THE ANTERIOR MANDIBULAR ARCH

The goals of oromandibular reconstruction include the restoration of form and function. Defects of the anterior mandibular arch, commonly referred to as Andy Gump deformities, produce a wide open mouth oriented towards the floor and are fortunately rarely seen today. This deformity is accompanied by loss of oral competence, excessive drooling, forfeiture of mastication, retropulsion of the tongue with speech impairment, and a notably morbid cosmetic deformity.

The superiority of vascularized osteocutaneous flaps for reconstruction of this defect has been well accepted for more than 3 decades. However, successful placement of vascularized bone and skin into these defects is often confused with successful reconstruction and rehabilitation. Truly successful reconstruction requires more nuanced

surgery than simple free tissue transfer. Careful preoperative evaluation of the volumes of the bone and soft tissue required needs to factor in, among many, one extremely important variable: the time elapsed since the bone was removed. The discontinuity created by the absence of the anterior mandibular arch leaves the proximal mandibular remnants at the mercy of traction from the muscles of mastication. These muscles pull the proximal remnants superiorly and medially and, after a few months, yield a forever-nonfunctional frozen temporomandibular joint complex (TMJ) with foreshortened, fibrosed muscles of mastication, even after the anterior mandible is replaced. The TMJ function associated with muscle fibrosis is made worse if the temporalis and pterygoid muscle connections to the mandible have been irradiated. This loss of function can be avoided by artificial maintenance of the mandibular arch after resection with external or internal fixation; but, unfortunately, many patients are months or years out from mandible loss without fixation when we meet. Without TMJ function, these patients will never have truly functional mandibles even after the best of bone and soft tissue replacement; their expectations need to be matched to this reality. However, even with tempered expectations, many patients are happy with any improvement in appearance or function. The other problem created by delayed replacement of the anterior arch is dramatic contraction and posterior displacement of the perioral, facial, and especially mental soft tissues. The resultant soft tissue defects will require replacement with soft tissue components of the donor flap, and resultant color mismatch will negatively impact the aesthetic outcome. Again, patient expectations need to be in line with reality.

Obviously, immediate reconstruction after anterior mandible loss is ideal; but for surgeons who inherit patients after months or years, the expectations will need to match achievable goals (**Fig. 4**).

- Prolonged mandibular discontinuity results in radical displacement of proximal mandibular remnants and fibrosis and permanent loss of function of the TMJs and muscles of mastication.
- Prolonged loss of anterior mandibular contour results in permanent contraction and distortion of the facial envelope of mouth lips and chin.
- Time to reconstruction is critical. Delayed reconstruction compromises functional and aesthetic outcomes. Immediate reconstruction is ideal.

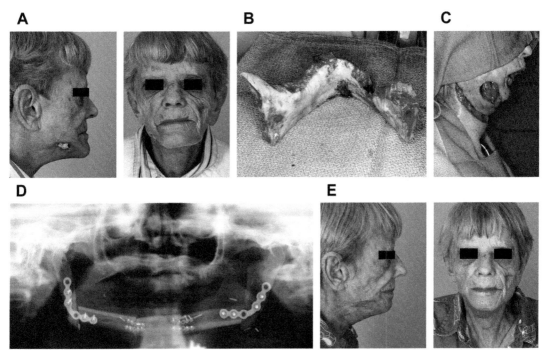

Fig. 4. Immediate reconstruction of anterior mandible defect. (*A*) Preoperative anterior and lateral view of a patient with ORN, demonstrating necrotic fractured mandible extruded from the right face. (*B*) Intraoperative view of subtotal mandibulectomy for widespread bilateral ORN. (*C*) Intraoperative lateral view of patient following mandibulectomy. The facial soft tissues are not supported and would contract dramatically if immediate reconstruction was not possible to support these soft tissues. (*D*) Postoperative panorex demonstrating fibula free flap reconstruction of the mandible. The patient had no prospects for osseointegration and dental rehabilitation, so the limited bone stock of the fibula needs to be used in such a way as to minimize the potential for a witch's profile. Note the superior orientation of the fibula bone away from the basilar aspect of the mandible. (*E*) Late (3 years) postoperative view, demonstrating the optimized appearance provided by the more superior location of the fibula. This location minimizes the posterior repositioning of the lower lip seen in reconstructed edentulous neomandibles when the fibula is placed at the basilar aspect of the mandible.

MANDIBLE RECONSTRUCTION AND OSSEOINTEGRATED IMPLANTS

Proper positioning of an osseus free flap for mandibular reconstruction ensures both a good functional and aesthetic outcome. The fibula, the favored first choice for mandible replacement, lacks the volume of native mandible. Please remember that the basilar aspect of the mandible does not approximate the dental arch. Anteriorly, this is particularly problematic; setting the bone in the plane of the outer cortex of the mental protuberance will result in an overly protruded mandible, made worse by the posterior collapse of the unsupported lower lip. If dental rehabilitation is planned, implants must, of course, be in the occlusal plane. This plane is posterior to the plane of the mental protuberance. Failure to correct for this results in an underbite and little or no labial-gingival sulcus anteriorly (**Fig. 5**).

We always ensure that the anterior mandible segment opposes the upper (maxillary) dental arch, which places the new bone many millimeters posterior to the original mental protuberance. We also double-barrel the fibula in the anterior segment to avoid inward posterior displacement of the lower lip, especially if patients are not candidates for osseointegrated implant dental rehabilitation. Our technique avoids large mandibular reconstruction bone plates anteriorly.

Also along the lateral mandibular arch, the basilar border of the mandible does not match the dental arch. The natural curve of the basilar bone is positioned lateral to the dental arch. We prefer a miniplate technique for mandible reconstruction as opposed to using a reconstructive bone plate. We create a template of the mandible in the occlusal plane. The neomandible can then be contoured and plated in a functional position. If patients are dentate and cancer precludes

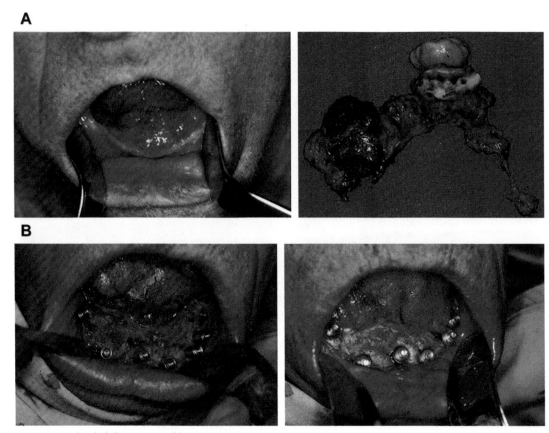

Fig. 5. Dental rehabilitation: problems created by placing the anterior mandible replacement at the basilar aspect of the mentum. (*A*) Intraoperative view demonstrating resection of anterior mandible, floor of mouth and anterior tongue with neck dissection. (*B*) Late postoperative dental office view of osseointegrated implants ready to be loaded with denture. Note the anterior location of this new dental arch which was anterior to the maxillary incisors producing an underbite. Note also the absence of a labial-gingival sulcus. This patient required revision surgery to retrodisplace his anterior mandible and achieve dental occlusion. This would have been unnecessary if the fibula reconstruction had not been positioned in the plane of the anterior mental protuberance.

contouring a plate over large portions of the mandible, the remaining teeth and mandible can be placed temporarily into maxillomandibular fixation before reconstruction in order to maintain occlusion. The interdental fixation is removed after the reconstruction is completed. If we do use a 3-dimensional model and a precontoured reconstructive mandibular bone plate in dentate patients, all but the proximal portion of that plate is removed after the fibula graft is properly positioned and fixed with small plates. When a lateral mandible segment is replaced, we prefer not to place the bone at the basilar aspect of the missing mandible for other reasons as well. Firstly, if implants are to be placed, the distance from the basilar aspect of the mandible to the dental occlusal surface is so long that cantilever forces on these implants might compromise outcomes. There is no reason to not position the fibula more

superiorly in the defect; the soft tissue paddle can be de-epithelialized and wrap the underside of the bone, restoring the basilar profile of the neomandible while ensuring that the bone is closer to the occlusal plane. Double-barreling the fibula can accomplish the same result.

Dental rehabilitation with osseointegrated implants has a success rate of more than 90%.[8–10] Timing of placement of osseointegrated implants is important in patients who will be receiving radiation. If postoperative RT is planned, it is recommended that the implants be placed at the time of surgery. It is generally considered that the success rate associated with the placement of osseointegrated implants in an already irradiated graft is lower.[8] These patients may have to go through a prolonged and more dangerous protocol for implants that may involve hyperbaric oxygen before the implants can be placed and loaded. If implants are placed at the time of the free flap reconstruction, there should be successful osseointegration before the time radiation is finished.

The heavily radiated facial soft tissue envelope atrophies. When a mandible needs replacement, this atrophic facial soft tissue envelope will scar to the bone flap of the underlying neomandible, producing an aesthetic and functional deformity. The neomandible is visible through the facial skin, and tethering produced by this scar inhibits facial expression at that site. This tethering can be avoided by sandwiching a de-epithelialized portion of the skin paddle used for intraoral repair between the facial soft tissues and the bone used for mandibular replacement.

- Avoid placement of fibula bone at the basilar aspect of the mandible.
- Successful mandibular reconstruction should include occlusal considerations. If dental rehabilitation is planned, the neomandible needs to be positioned in the occlusal plane.
- We prefer to place osseointegrated implants at the time of free tissue transfer in patients who will receive adjuvant RT to maximize the success of osseointegration.
- De-epithelialized flap skin between the mandibular reconstruction and radiated atrophied facial skin envelope improves appearance and facial expression.

TRISMUS

Trismus can be one of the most unfavorable functional outcomes of head and neck cancer treatment. Consequences of poor mouth opening include poor oral hygiene, difficult tumor surveillance, limitation to oral intake, speech difficulties, and ultimate loss of teeth.

Several mouth-opening measurements have been used to define trismus. A mouth opening of 35 mm or less is a reasonable functional cutoff for defining trismus in head and neck patient populations.[11] We have learned that trismus is primarily a result of radiation effect over time on the muscles of mastication. Exercises include active range-of-motion exercises, hold-relax techniques, and manual stretching.[11–13] Despite exercise therapy, trismus can be difficult to reverse or combat.[12] We frequently have to perform brisement procedures and coronoidectomies.

Adequate mouth opening and mastication depends on a functional temporomandibular joint. Even if malignancies of the oral cavity or ORN of the mandible do not directly involve the condyle, superior surgical resection may leave an inadequate condylar segment for plate fixation. Many options have been outlined for reconstructing the condyle: use of a condylar prosthesis, securing the nonvascular residual condyle to the end of the fibula, and directly placing the distal fibula into the glenoid fossa.[14,15] The use of condylar prosthesis has largely been abandoned for mandibular reconstruction because of fears of erosion through the glenoid fossa into the middle fossa. We prefer not to use nonvascularized condylar bone, fearing avascular necrosis, especially if patients are to receive RT. Our reconstructive method of choice is to place the distal fibula directly into the joint. The distal fibula bone is contoured round, and a hole is drilled at the distal most end through which a permanent suture is threaded. This suture is then loosely secured to the remaining joint capsule and bone of the glenoid fossa. This placement minimizes lateral excursion of the neocondyle on mouth opening. A true sliding hinge joint is impossible to reconstruct. In order to best ensure that temporofibular ankylosis does not occur, we recommend designing the fibula skin paddle long enough so that the end of the skin paddle can be de-epithelized and placed between the distal fibula bone and joint capsule (**Fig. 6**).

- Trismus can compromise the function of a successful head and neck reconstruction. Management includes exercise therapy and may require brisement procedures to increase mouth opening.
- When reconstructing mandibular defects involving the condyle, we favor loosely securing the distal bone graft to the glenoid fossa, preserving the superior articular cartilage of the joint when possible. De-epithelialized skin paddle can be inserted in between the bone and capsule to help avoid ankylosis.

HAIR-BEARING FLAPS

Many free flap donor sites are hair bearing in contrast to the mucosa of the upper aerodigestive tract. Intraoral and pharyngeal hairy flaps can be an annoyance. This problem is not an issue if patients are going to receive postoperative RT because radiation kills hair follicles. If RT is not planned, these flaps will need to be depilated later. This procedure can be done easily with monopolar cautery or laser in an office setting for oral defects but usually requires sedation for repairs of the lower oropharynx and hypopharynx. Not only should hair-bearing skin never be placed in the nasal cavity but also skin itself should never be

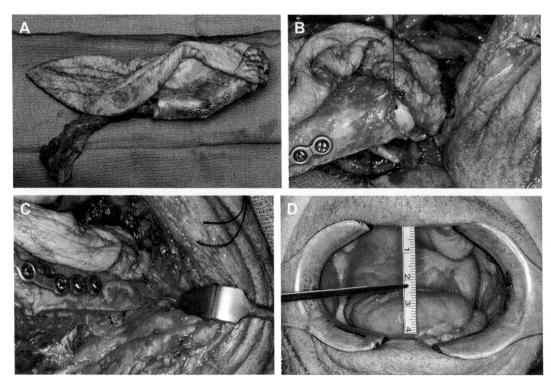

Fig. 6. Avoidance of ankylosis of reconstructed temporomandibular pseudojoint. (*A*) Intraoperative view demonstrating fibula flap construct for replacement of left mandible body and ramus including condyle. Note position of the fibula skin flap destined for de-epithelialization and its orientation to the fibula condyle replacement. The remainder of the fibula skin paddle will reconstruct the intraoral soft tissue defect. (*B*) Intraoperative view demonstrating the de-epithelialized fibula skin sandwiched between the glenoid fossa and the bone. Note polypropylene (Prolene) suture that will anchor this fibula to the glenoid fossa. (*C*) Intraoperative view demonstrating the new joint. (*D*) Late postoperative view demonstrating the excellent excursion (mouth opening) presented by this maneuver.

used to line the sinonasal cavity as it will produce odiferous mucous crusts. We only use muscle or de-epithelialized skin paddles to line the sinonasal cavities. These surfaces will then remucosalize and not produce such crusting.

PHARYNGOESOPHAGEAL RECONSTRUCTION

Pharyngoesophageal defects most commonly result from oncologic resections of malignancies of the larynx and hypopharynx. However, in the era of CXRT for head and neck cancer, delayed stenosis and even obliteration of the pharynx or esophagus from radiation has become a growing problem. These patients have additional considerations regarding functional outcomes, namely swallowing. Despite a worthy reconstruction the effects of radiation continue. The reconstructed neopharynx or the adjacent pharyngoesophagus is more likely to restenose in this population of over-radiated patients than in reconstructions performed after primary oncologic pharyngoesophagectomy. We recommend overcorrection. When using free

fasciocutaneous flaps, namely, the radial forearm and anterolateral thigh flaps, we recommend the lock-and-key technique. The concept was first introduced in the 1980s by the senior author (REH) to minimize contraction and stenosis of the circular suture lines.[16–18] A triangular-shaped extension (key) is designed in the distal skin paddle that locks into an opposing linear incision in the cervical esophagus, which breaks up the vectors of contraction, minimizing stenosis.

If a jejunal segment is used to reconstruct this defect, the segment of jejunum harvested needs to closely match the length of the pharyngoesophageal defect (**Fig. 7**). Put the jejunum on stretch before harvest for accurate measurement, and tack a suture to the serosa to indicate which end is distal so that the reconstructed segment will not cause dysphagia secondary to retrograde peristalsis.

One of the most unfavorable situations encountered in total pharyngoesophageal reconstruction after radiation is failure of the well-vascularized tubed skin flap to heal to the adjacent over-radiated pharynx and esophagus. In a small

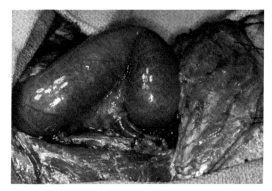

Fig. 7. Necessity of accurate measurement of donor length of jejunum. Intraoperative view demonstrating the senior author's first jejunal transfer for reconstruction of a pharyngoesophageal defect. Note the contracted (unmeasured) jejunal segment seemed to be identical to the length of the defect until revascularized. The segment then regained its preharvest length and had to be significantly shortened to avoid severe dysphagia.

number of cases, this dehiscence and resultant fistula can be significant enough to warrant conversion to a 2-stage reconstruction. These circumstances necessitate externalization of the flap. The flap is secured to the posterior pharyngeal and esophageal walls thereby creating pharyngostoma and esophagostoma. The tubed flap is untubed and used to cover the great vessels. After healing has occurred, a second procedure with a second flap is required to reconstruct the pharyngeal conduit.

TOTAL GLOSSECTOMY RECONSTRUCTION

Before free tissue transfer, total glossectomy required a total laryngectomy to avoid recurrent aspiration pneumonia and its associated morbidity and mortality. Early attempts to preserve the larynx after total glossectomy unsuccessfully used the pectoralis major myocutaneous pedicled flap. Following reconstruction of the tongue with the pectoralis flap, the denervated pectoralis muscle would atrophy, within the oral cavity, exposing the larynx to unprotected aspiration (**Fig. 8**).

The senior author first used the reinnervated latissimus dorsi musculocutaneous flap in 1984 to reconstruct total glossectomy defects while preserving the larynx.[19]

Our techniques have evolved since then to include the many free tissue options available, including the rectus abdominis myocutaneous flap, latissimus dorsi myocutaneous flap, radial forearm fasciocutaneous flap, anterolateral thigh fasciocutaneous flap, and the parascapular or transverse scapular fasciocutaneous flaps. Functional outcomes are respectable. Tracheotomy decannulation rates vary between 85% and 95%, whereas gastrostomy tube dependency ranges from 30% to 44%.[20–23]

For reconstruction of the neotongue, maintenance of tissue bulk maximizes speech. Revascularized denervated muscle atrophies. Revascularized and reinnervated muscle will maintain bulk, but any motion that is restored does not replicate that of a normal tongue and has questionable contribution to speech and swallowing. Revascularized fat and dermis undergoes minimal atrophy and is ideal to maintain the needed bulk for function. Therefore, we now favor the use of fasciocutaneous free flaps for total tongue reconstruction. Our workhorse fasciocutaneous flaps for this purpose are the anterolateral thigh flap and parascapular flap, both of which can be harvested with very large skin paddles. The large skin paddles of the flap are not wasted, rather much of the skin is de-epithelized and rolled under itself to increase the soft tissue bulk of the neotongue. At the conclusion of the reconstruction, the neotongue should ideally contact the palate. As perioperative swelling resides, the tissue will

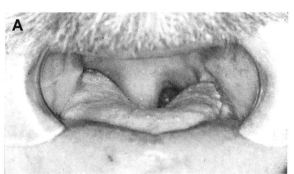
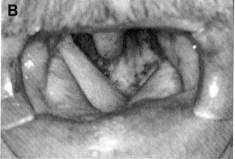

Fig. 8. Early attempt at total glossectomy reconstruction with pectoralis major pedicled flap. (*A*) Early postoperative view of pectoralis flap in the mouth. (*B*) Late (6 months) postoperative view demonstrating atrophy of the denervated muscle and loss of oral cavity bulk.

lose some size but should maintain enough bulk for good speech (**Fig. 9**).

An important lesson learned during total glossectomy reconstruction is to create a platform for suspension of the soft tissue of the neotongue. Without suspension, caudal migration of the neotongue through the mandibular arch into the anterior neck results in inadequate bulk in the oral cavity. There are 2 technical considerations we use to avoid this. First, if harvesting the anterolateral thigh flap, we include large fascial wings that extend beyond the skin paddle. Drill holes in the mandible are used to secure the fascia and create a suspension on which sits the fat, de-epithelialized flap and skin of the neotongue. Second, if a parascapular flap is used, we often harvest both the parascapular and transverse scapular skin paddles, using one paddle to span the mandibular arch and the remaining skin paddle to build on this platform. Likewise, a composite scapular flap with either the lateral border or scapular tip can be harvested. The bone can be plated across the mandibular arch to support the skin paddle in the oral cavity.

Suspension of the larynx maximizes swallowing. By suspending the hyoid bone to the anterior mandibular arch, the larynx is repositioned in a more anterior and superior position, ideal for swallowing and preventing aspiration.

Even with total glossectomy and total laryngectomy, we think an effort should be made to reconstruct the tongue. Although speech is more severely compromised with both total laryngectomy and total glossectomy, we have several patients who are able to successfully communicate with understandable speech using tracheoesophageal speech and a reconstructed neotongue.

- Revascularized denervated muscle atrophies. Revascularized reinnervated muscle and revascularized fat and dermis will not atrophy and will maintain tissue bulk for reasonable speech.

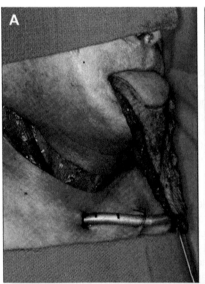
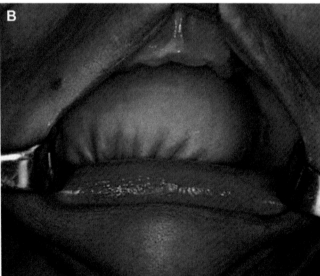
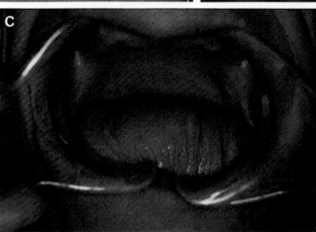

Fig. 9. Total glossectomy reconstruction with free latissimus dorsi flap. (*A*) Intraoperative view of the vascular anastomoses and nerve anastomosis of the thoracodorsal nerve to the remnant proximal hypoglossal nerve. (*B*) Donor site result. (*C*) Early postoperative view (*left*) and late (7 years) (*right*) view. Note the minimal atrophy over several years of the revascularized reinnervated muscle.

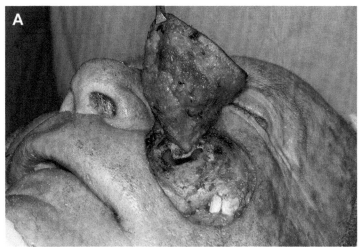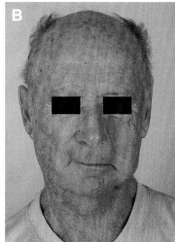

Fig. 10. Color match of the submental flap to facial skin. (*A*) Intraoperative view of skin cancer resection involving left face and anterior maxilla. (*B*) Late postoperative view demonstrates a good color match of the submental skin paddle to the face.

- The bulk of the neotongue should contact the palate at conclusion of surgery as some settling always occurs. Support the oral soft tissue with suspension techniques to prevent descent into the neck, compromising the bulk in the oral cavity.
- Bulk of the neotongue maximizes speech.
- Suspension of the larynx maximizes swallowing.
- Even in total glossectomy with total laryngectomy, tongue reconstruction allows for compromised yet functional tracheoesophageal speech.

SUBMENTAL FLAP: IDEAL COLOR MATCH FOR FACIAL RECONSTRUCTION

Our frustration with the poor color match provided by remote free flaps for reconstruction of facial defects has caused us to use an increasing number of submental pedicled, hybrid, or free flaps.[24–27] The color match and hair-bearing qualities of this donor site are unrivalled for facial reconstruction (**Fig. 10**).

REFERENCES

1. Suh JD, Sercarz JA, Abemayor E, et al. Analysis of outcome and complications in 400 cases of microvascular head and neck reconstruction. Arch Otolaryngol Head Neck Surg 2004;130(8):962–6.
2. Nakatsuka T, Harii K, Asato H, et al. Analytic review of 2372 free flap transfers for head and neck reconstruction following cancer resection. J Reconstr Microsurg 2003;19(6):363–8 [discussion: 369].
3. Urken ML, Weinberg H, Buchbinder D, et al. Microvascular free flaps in head and neck reconstruction. Report of 200 cases and review of complications. Arch Otolaryngol Head Neck Surg 1994;120(6): 633–40.
4. Smith DJ. Effects of gamma radiation on isolated surviving arteries and their vasa vasorum. Am J Physiol 1961;201:901–4.
5. Oh JC, Weber RS, Bagley LJ, et al. Ruptured pseudoaneurysm of the internal maxillary artery complicating CT-guided fine-needle aspiration in an irradiated, surgical bed. Head Neck 2007;29(12):1156–9.
6. Nagel TH, Howard BE, Donald CB, et al. Recipient artery rupture in free tissue transfer in heavily radiated beds. AAO-HNSF Annual Meeting. Vancouver, British Columbia, Canada, September 29, 2013.
7. Hayden RE, Kirby SD, Deschler DG. Technical modifications of the latissimus dorsi pedicled flap to increase versatility and viability. Laryngoscope 2000; 110(3 Pt 1):352–7.
8. Barber HD, Seckinger RJ, Hayden RE, et al. Evaluation of osseointegration of endosseous implants in radiated, vascularized fibula flaps to the mandible: a pilot study. J Oral Maxillofac Surg 1995;53(6): 640–4 [discussion: 644–5].
9. Urken ML, Buchbinder D, Weinberg H, et al. Primary placement of osseointegrated implants in microvascular mandibular reconstruction. Otolaryngol Head Neck Surg 1989;101(1):56–73.
10. Urken ML, Buchbinder D, Costantino PD, et al. Oromandibular reconstruction using microvascular composite flaps: report of 210 cases. Arch Otolaryngol Head Neck Surg 1998;124(1):46–55.
11. Dijkstra PU, Kalk WW, Roodenburg JL. Trismus in head and neck oncology: a systematic review. Oral Oncol 2004;40(9):879–89.
12. Dijkstra PU, Sterken MW, Pater R, et al. Exercise therapy for trismus in head and neck cancer. Oral Oncol 2007;43(4):389–94.

13. Cohen EG, Deschler DG, Walsh K, et al. Early use of a mechanical stretching device to improve mandibular mobility after composite resection: a pilot study. Arch Phys Med Rehabil 2005;86(7):1416–9.

14. Guyot L, Richard O, Layoun W, et al. Long-term radiological findings following reconstruction of the condyle with fibular free flaps. J Craniomaxillofac Surg 2004;32(2):98–102.

15. Wax MK, Winslow CP, Hansen J, et al. A retrospective analysis of temporomandibular joint reconstruction with free fibula microvascular flap. Laryngoscope 2000;110(6):977–81.

16. Hayden RE. Lateral thigh free flaps for reconstruction of total laryngopharyngectomy defects. Joint meeting SHNS and ASHNS. Baltimore, MD, 1984.

17. Hayden RE. A new technique for pharyngoesophageal reconstruction. In: Bloom HJG, editor. Head and neck oncology. New York: Raven Press; 1986. p. 127–35.

18. Hayden RE. Reconstruction of the hypopharynx and cervical esophagus. In: Cummings CC, editor. Otolaryngology – head and neck surgery. St Louis (MO): Mosby; 1993. p. 2186–97.

19. Hayden RE, Fredrickson JM. A new technique for reconstruction after total glossectomy. Joint meeting SHNS and ASHNS. San Juan, PR, 1985.

20. Rigby MH, Hayden RE. Total glossectomy without laryngectomy - a review of functional outcomes and reconstructive principles. Curr Opin Otolaryngol Head Neck Surg 2014;22(5):414–8.

21. Rihani J, Lee MR, Lee T, et al. Flap selection and functional outcomes in total glossectomy with laryngeal preservation. Otolaryngol Head Neck Surg 2013;149(4):547–53.

22. Dziegielewski PT, Ho ML, Rieger J, et al. Total glossectomy with laryngeal preservation and free flap reconstruction: objective functional outcomes and systematic review of the literature. Laryngoscope 2013;123(1):140–5.

23. Navach V, Zurlo V, Calabrese L, et al. Total glossectomy with preservation of the larynx: oncological and functional results. Br J Oral Maxillofac Surg 2013;51(3):217–23.

24. Martin D, Pascal JF, Baudet J, et al. The submental island flap: a new donor site. Anatomy and clinical applications as a free or pedicled flap. Plast Reconstr Surg 1993;92:867–73.

25. Patel UA, Bayles SW, Hayden RE. The submental flap: a modified technique for resident training. Laryngoscope 2007;117:186–9.

26. Rigby MH, Hayden RE. Regional flaps: a move to simpler reconstructive options in the head and neck. Curr Opin Otolaryngol Head Neck Surg 2014;22(5):401–6.

27. Hayden RE, Nagel TH, Donald CB. Hybrid submental flaps for reconstruction in the head and neck: part pedicled, part free. Laryngoscope 2014;124(3):637–41.

Unfavorable Results After Free Tissue Transfer to Head and Neck

Lessons Learned at the University of Washington

Jeffrey J. Houlton, MD*, Scott E. Bevans, MD, Neal D. Futran, MD

KEYWORDS

- Free flap reconstruction • Free tissue transfer • Antibiotics • Tracheotomy tube placement
- Total glossectomy • Laryngopharyngectomy • Total cervical esophagectomy • Jejunal free flap

KEY POINTS

- Overnight intubation has allowed a decrease in the use of tracheotomy tube placement without adverse patient outcomes. The authors have found earlier return to normal swallow, decreased intensive care unit stay duration, and decreased overall hospitalization.
- Current practice is to follow the Infectious Disease Society of America guidelines for perioperative antibiotic use with ampicillin-sulbactam or clindamycin with levofloxacin (or another agent for broad-spectrum gram-negative coverage) for 24 hours postoperatively.
- For postoperative flap monitoring, the authors use a needle-stick technique every 6 hours for 72 hours postoperatively. For buried flaps without a monitor paddle, the authors use both arterial and venous Cook implantable Dopplers.
- For total glossectomy defects, our preference has evolved to use the anterolateral thigh flap for its bulk, minimal atrophy, and large surface area. We use the fascia of the vastus lateralis to suspend the flap to the mandible and perform hyoid suspension concomitantly.
- For total cervical esophagectomy defects, our preference is to use jejunal free flap secondary to improved swallow outcomes with decreased fistula and stricture rates. We have found the voice changes to be inconsequential to patients.

INTRODUCTION

Free tissue transfer to the head and neck is a complex and multistep procedure. With experience, clinicians can become proficient with the reconstructive technique, but achieving consistently reliable functional and cosmetic results is a challenge even for the most seasoned surgeon, particularly when reconstructing head and neck oncologic defects, which are frequently seen in previously irradiated patients with complex functional needs and/or multiple medical comorbid conditions.

At the University of Washington (UW), the senior author has performed more than 2500 free tissue

Disclosures: J.J. Houlton and N.D. Futran have no disclosures to report. S.E. Bevans (MAJ, MC) is a member of the United States Army. The views expressed herein are those of the authors and do not reflect the official policy or position of the Department of the Army, Department of Defense, or the US government.
Department of Otolaryngology, University of Washington, 1959 Northeast Pacific Street, Box 356515, Seattle, WA 98195, USA
* Corresponding author.
E-mail address: jhoulton@uw.edu

Clin Plastic Surg 43 (2016) 683–693
http://dx.doi.org/10.1016/j.cps.2016.05.006

transfers to the head and neck over the past 20 years. This article shares our experience with 3 areas that we find particularly challenging in the management of our patients. The article describes our approach to postoperative care, because most unfavorable outcomes arise in the early postoperative period. It then describes 2 complicated defects: the total glossectomy defect and the total laryngopharyngectomy defect. These 2 defects result in severe form and functional losses for patients and are challenging to adequately restore.

POSTOPERATIVE MANAGEMENT: MINIMIZING THE MORBIDITY OF HEAD AND NECK FREE FLAP SURGERY

Convalescence from head and neck free flap surgery is a challenging endeavor. Recent studies suggest that between 11% and 52% of patients with head and neck cancer meet Diagnostic and Statistical Manual of Mental Disorders criteria for major depressive disorder during treatment and recovery.[1–4] As a result, some recent investigators have suggested the prophylactic initiation of antidepressant therapy for all patients with head and neck cancer[5] because of the common and significant physiologic insults caused by either surgery or postoperative chemoradiotherapy. In the postoperative period, significant facial/neck swelling, restriction of oral intake, loss of normal vocalization, frequent blood draws, and invasive procedures contribute to a high rate of discomfort and, at times, hopelessness. In addition to the development of a free flap clinical care pathway, the authors have focused on 3 aspects of postoperative management that, in our experience, have minimized morbidity and improved the quality of care: reduction in tracheostomy tube placement, prevention of postoperative infection while minimizing side effects and complications associated with antibiotic use, and reduction in the risk of free flap loss with dependable monitoring.

Development of a Clinical Care Pathway

The perioperative care of all free flap patients at UW is guided by a streamlined clinical care pathway. This pathway begins preoperatively with significant counseling and an assessment of anticipated postoperative social work/nursing needs. Our head and neck cancer care team consents patient before surgery for peripherally inserted central catheter (PICC) and percutaneous endoscopic gastrostomy (PEG) placement; procedures that are performed while the patient is still anesthetized in the intensive care unit (ICU) the morning after surgery. PEG placement ensures that patients receive enteral tube feeds and

medications within 24 hours of surgery, allowing the decreased use of intravenous fluids and avoiding the discomfort of a nasal tube. The PICC allows most new needle sticks to be avoided during their stay. Although these measures do not eliminate the recovery burden, anecdotally, they make the hospitalization and immediate home care much more tolerable. In addition, early ambulation and care by a focused head and neck nursing team has resulted in a 2-day reduction of hospital stay (average now 8.2 days) and increased levels of patient satisfaction within the first 6 months of implementation of the care pathway.

Overnight Intubation Versus Tracheostomy

Tracheostomy has traditionally been considered the mainstay of airway management following free tissue transfer to the head and neck. Many patients require this type of secure airway to avoid life-threatening obstruction; however, tracheostomy tube placement involves morbidity and complications. Therefore, at UW, we have shifted the airway management paradigm to reduce tracheostomy-related morbidity by avoiding tracheostomy in most of our head and neck free flap patients.

Tracheostomy tube complications include bleeding, infection, mucous plugging, tracheitis, aspiration-related pneumonia, and tracheal stenosis.[6] Data suggest that there may be an increased risk of pulmonary complications in head and neck patients with tracheostomies, because tracheostomy is known to exacerbate aspiration, although it does improve pulmonary toilet.[7,8] Avoiding a tracheostomy allows patients to speak earlier and maintain a strong cough. A tracheostomy may require increased nursing care and patient education and frequently complicates patients' placement after surgery, because many US skilled nursing facilities are disinclined to approve the transfer of patients with tracheostomy tubes.

In a 2010 retrospective review published by our UW group, 37 patients who were nasally intubated following an oral cavity resection/free flap reconstructions were compared with 21 patients who underwent a tracheostomy following similar oral cavity reconstruction.[9] The mean hospital stay (8.4 days vs 12.4 days) and the likelihood of requiring a feeding tube (19% vs 76%) at discharge were both independently increased in the tracheostomy group on multivariate analysis. There were no airway emergencies or secondary tracheostomies performed in the nasal intubation group.

Similarly, there seems to be a growing trend elsewhere in the literature toward the decreased use of tracheostomy tubes in patients undergoing head and neck free tissue transfer. In a 2014 report by Moubayed and colleagues,[10] 66 patients underwent mandibulectomy with osteocutaneous free flap reconstruction without tracheostomy. There were no deaths or major safety events in the series, although 1 patient required an urgent secondary tracheostomy and 2 patients reported airway obstructive symptoms. A 2013 study by Coyle and colleagues[8] reported outcomes of 50 patients undergoing free flap reconstruction with oncologic resections without a tracheostomy and a similar group of 50 patients who underwent an elective tracheostomy. There were no airway emergencies or secondary tracheostomies reported in the intubation group. In addition, the intubation group had a shorter ICU stay (1.4 days vs 3.7 days), shorter overall hospital stay (13 days vs 18 days), and a lower rate of pneumonia (10% vs 38%).

Since our 2010 publication, it has become our preference to avoid a tracheostomy in most patients undergoing free flap reconstruction. Defects for which we prefer overnight intubation include most defects of the oral cavity: large reconstructions of the oral tongue, and lateral and anterior floor of mouth; segmental mandibulectomy; as well as maxillectomy, external skin, skull base, or parotidectomy defects. Patients who we think will still benefit from an elective tracheostomy include patients who require free tissue transfer for total glossectomy defects, oropharyngeal defects (both pharyngeal and base of tongue), and hypopharyngeal defects. We are also prone to consider a tracheostomy in patients with very poor lung function, trismus, and bulky flaps that would significantly complicate reintubation. If the ease of reintubation is in question, we frequently assess laryngeal exposure with a postoperative direct laryngoscopy before the patient leaves the operating room.

Patients for whom a tracheostomy is deferred receive intravenous steroids (Decadron 10 mg intravenously every 8 hours for 24 hours) while in the ICU overnight, and then they are extubated on the first postoperative morning, unless significant airway swelling has developed. Using this approach, only a very few patients have required further airway management.

Postoperative Infections

One important clinical challenge following head and neck free tissue transfer is the high rate of postoperative infections. The location and nature of head and neck cancer resection often directly violates oral/pharyngeal surfaces and thus exposes wounds to a significant bacterial burden.

This exposure places patients at high risk of wound infection, with an incidence of 8% to 45%.[11] Limiting the rate of infection is critical in free flap surgery, because infection increases the risk of wound complications and microvascular failure. However, a consensus on the type and duration of antibiotic prophylaxis has not been uniformly established. In a landmark 1984 study, Johnson and colleagues[12] reported that the rate of infection following head and neck cancer surgery, which was highest in oropharyngeal resections and free flap reconstructions, was greatly reduced by treating patients with 5 days of postoperative clindamycin and gentamicin (broad-spectrum gram-positive/gram-negative coverage). In 2014, the same author performed a literature review and proposed evidence-based recommendations for treatment with 24 hours of perioperative antibiotic therapy for clean-contaminated head and neck surgery.[13] This proposal is consistent with current guidelines from the Infectious Disease Society of America (IDSA), Surgical Infection Society, and Society for Healthcare Epidemiology of America, all of which recommend 24 hours of antibiotic prophylaxis for major clean-contaminated procedures.[14]

The authors recently analyzed and published changes to our prophylactic antibiotic protocol for patients undergoing head and neck free tissue transfer procedures.[15] As we transitioned from prolonged courses of antibiotics, as Johnson and colleagues initially published, to the IDSA-recommended 24-hour duration, our data showed that within 30 days of surgery (which is the US Centers for Disease Control and Prevention defined time period for surgical site infection) 45% of the patients were treated for at least 1 infection: 22% at the flap inset site, 12% at donor site, and 17% at any other site (eg, pneumonia, urinary tract infection). The rate of infection in patients who received 24 hours of antibiotics was higher at 57% compared with a 42% rate in patients who received prolonged courses of antibiotics (most commonly 7 days) after surgery (P = .01). Use of clindamycin alone relative to ampicillin-sulbactam increased the risk of postoperative infection (odds ratio [OR], 2.5; P = .01), which is presumably from limiting gram-negative bacterial coverage in patients who received clindamycin alone. In multivariate analysis, the other factor most strongly associated with postoperative infection was hypothyroidism (OR, 10.8; P<.001).

Some of these findings are in conflict with other recent studies, including a 2015 study by Khariwala and colleagues[16] showing an increased rate of pneumonia in patients receiving longer courses of antibiotics with no reduction in surgical site infection in patients undergoing radial forearm flap reconstruction following a laryngectomy. In their analysis, obesity was the greatest risk factor and had the highest OR for developing a postoperative infection.

Postoperative antibiotic use does involve harm. The increasing frequency of antibiotic-associated complications (eg, drug reactions, *Clostridium difficile* infections), as well as the emergence of increasing multidrug-resistant bacteria, are intuitive reasons to avoid prolonged courses of antimicrobial therapy. However, recent data on the duration of perioperative antibiotic use are sparse in the head and neck free flap population. In our study, there was no clear correlation between antibiotic duration and *C difficile* infection or multidrug-resistant infection. However, this may be institutionally dependent.

In conclusion, data from our institution show a high rate of infection following head and neck free flap surgery despite adherence to the IDSA perioperative guidelines. Contributing to this high rate may be our inclusion of the full 30-day observation period, or it may represent our bias toward having a very low threshold for diagnosing postoperative infection and initiating treatment. Despite this result, our current preference is to adhere to the shorter IDSA-recommended 24 hours of broad-spectrum antimicrobial prophylaxis using ampicillin-sulbactam (first line) or clindamycin/levofloxacin (for gram-negative bacteria coverage) in patients with ampicillin allergy. The authors continue to maintain a very low threshold for prolonged antibiotic use (5 to 7 days) for patients with hypothyroidism or poor wound healing given supportive data from our recent report.

Postoperative Free Flap Monitoring

More than 20 different methods for free flap monitoring have been described in the literature.[17] Methods range from a simple clinical examination and pinprick testing to using complex technological innovations, including methods using implantable Doppler ultrasonography, microdialysis probes, oxygen saturation probes, laser Doppler, fluorometry, implantable temperature probes, glucose/lactate monitors, handheld Doppler, scintigraphy, pH monitoring, impedance plethysmography, confocal microscopy, smartphone serial photoimaging, and several other techniques.

Despite this variety, the goals of monitoring remain singularly focused on reducing the rate of free flap loss. Monitoring techniques achieve this goal by heralding the risk of free flap compromise before overt clinical change, thus improving the chances of free flap salvage. Timely identification of a threatened flap increases the rate of salvage

and decreases the risk of the no-reflow phenomenon.[18]

Despite a high rate of free flap survival, clinicians at UW continue to place a high priority on meticulous monitoring to ensure our high rate of success. Over the past 20 years, many methods for free flap monitoring have been tried by the authors, but in our practice no method has been as reliable and accurate as simple skin prick testing. Our protocol calls for a nursing-performed clinical examination every hour for the first 24 hours while patients are in the ICU overnight. In addition, the flap is checked by a physician with a clinical examination and pinprick testing every 6 hours for a total of 72 hours. After 72 hours, the flap is checked twice daily without planned pinprick until discharge.

In order to facilitate pinprick monitoring, a concerted effort is made to develop a monitoring paddle during reconstruction. If a monitoring paddle is not used (a completely buried flap), then we use an implantable Doppler system on both the artery and the venous outflow. This use of the Cook implantable Doppler on buried flaps has been shown to be particularly valuable, as was shown in a 2011 retrospective review of 548 microsurgical cases in which the rate of salvage for buried flaps was improved significantly with use of the implantable Doppler versus a clinical examination alone (94% vs 40%).[19] Continuous implantable Dopplers are also preferred following free flap take-backs that require revision of the microvascular anastomosis.

Fig. 1 shows the use of pinprick testing with a 25-gauge needle. A reassuring result is shown by the delayed (2 to 5 seconds) appearance of bright red blood. **Fig. 2** shows a flap that is congested on pinprick testing. The 46-year-old patient underwent a composite oral cavity resection followed by reconstruction with an osteocutaneous radial forearm flap. On the first postoperative day, the patient was noted as having dark venous blood on pinprick testing. A subsequent take-back was significant for

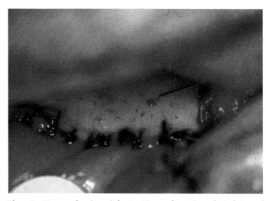

Fig. 1. Normal pinprick testing showing bright red blood following needle stick.

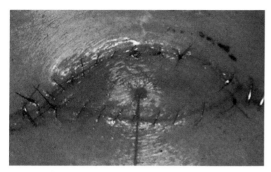

Fig. 2. Abnormal pinprick testing showing dark red blood indicates venous congestion.

the twisting of the venous outflow tract causing venous obstruction. A revision venous anastomosis was performed and no further issues developed, resulting in successful free flap salvage.

Using the pinprick method with judicious use of the implantable Doppler has generally yielded a high rate of free flap success and salvage. A review of an unpublished personal database by the senior author (NDF) reveals an overall flap success rate of 99.2% in 2734 free flaps. The corresponding take-back rate is 4.1% with a salvage rate of 91%. There is a partial flap necrosis rate of 6.6%.

LESSON LEARNED FROM RECONSTRUCTION OF THE TOTAL GLOSSECTOMY DEFECT

The total glossectomy defect (with the preservation of the larynx) represents one of our most significant reconstructive challenges. Loss of tongue function, even with adequate tissue restoration, is a serious consequence for patients, resulting in a propensity for aspiration as well as distortion of articulation and swallowing. A total glossectomy is generally performed in patients who are severely malnourished and often previously irradiated (oropharyngeal). Loss of flap bulk and the lack of long-term suspension of the neotongue frequently diminish long-term reconstructive results. This loss of neotongue volume has repeatedly been shown to result in poorer swallowing and voice outcomes.[20–22]

The appropriateness of a total glossectomy with laryngeal preservation was controversial until the 1980s to 1990s.[23,24] Before this, controversy existed as to whether head and neck surgeons should perform concurrent total laryngectomy in all patients undergoing a total glossectomy because of concerns of poor residual laryngeal function. Before the widespread advent of free tissue transfer, total glossectomy defects were generally reconstructed with the pectoralis flap. This flap had a significant issue with maintaining bulk in the oral cavity and frequently receded into

the neck with gravity during recovery and atrophy. Swallowing results were poor and many patients were left with an essentially nonfunctional larynx (if laryngeal preservation was attempted). The evolution toward improved free tissue reconstructive techniques has decreased the need for total laryngectomy. Despite these reconstruction improvements, patients remain at a high risk for severe dysphagia, aspiration, and poor articulation.

In theory, the ideal flap choice for reconstructing the total glossectomy defect would be designed with significant oversized bulk, would not atrophy significantly over time, and would remain suspended in the oral cavity. Flap bulk is critical to the oral phase of swallowing. In order to maintain a functional oral swallow, the neotongue must remain in contact with the palate to allow the patient to maintain an adequate suction with oral swallowing. This palatal contact requires that the flap not undergo a significant loss of bulk and maintains adequate suspension. In addition, it is necessary to have significant oropharyngeal/base of tongue bulk to divert the food/liquid bolus away from the glottis during the oropharyngeal phase of swallowing, rather than funneling the bolus toward the laryngeal inlet, which is frequently associated with undersized flaps.

In our experience, the radial forearm and lateral arm free flaps do not maintain enough bulk to achieve the volume needed for the neotongue. **Fig. 3** shows lack of bulk following lateral arm free flap reconstruction of a total oral tongue defect. The rectus abdominis and latissimus dorsi free flaps are more appropriate choices, capable of the necessary volume recreation. However, we

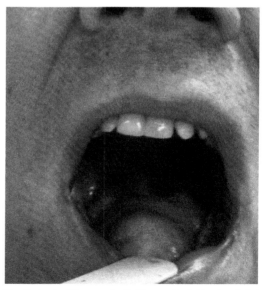

Fig. 3. Lack of tongue bulk 12 months following total glossectomy reconstruction with a lateral arm flap.

have found that, given their significant muscle bulk, they tend to atrophy significantly with time. These flaps are secondary choices in our practice. Our first choice of a free flap donor site is the anterolateral thigh (in patients with suitable subcutaneous tissue of the upper leg). This flap is typically ideal because it has significant adipose tissue, a strong fascial layer from the vastus lateralis for suspension, and a muscular cuff that can be harvested to provide additional bulk.

The following patient presentation represents our general approach to the total glossectomy defect and the most important concepts to avoid poor outcomes following total glossectomy.

Patient Presentation: Reconstruction of the Total Glossectomy Defect

A 45-year-old man presented with a recurrent large oral cavity cancer, with history of prior chemoradiation therapy, invading both the complete oral cavity as well as the base of tongue. **Fig. 4** shows the resulting total glossectomy defect, with complete resection of the base of tongue. When approaching this type of defect, it is important to attempt to preserve some functional base of the tongue during the oncologic procedure. Ideally, the base of preserved tongue should have some sensory input from the glossopharyngeal or lingual nerves and some motor input via branches of the hypoglossal nerve. If this is not oncologically possible, a complete total glossectomy is performed. However, a near-total glossectomy, in our experience, results in better

functional restoration. We approach this resection via a visor flap and pull-through technique as opposed to a lip split and mandibular split approach. Access to the tumor is equal in both approaches, but we avoid potential bone healing complications, issues with wound breakdown in the buccal sulcus, and unsightly facial scarring.

A flap donor site with significant adipose tissue is chosen. Our first preference is the anterolateral thigh (ALT) flap. If the thigh is a poor donor site because of a cachexia or aberrant vasculature, then our secondary choice is the latissimus dorsi or rectus abdominis free flap.

The ALT flap is harvested in a fairly standard fashion. The skin paddle is intentionally oversized, with its width approximated by measuring the distance from molar to contralateral molar in a curvilinear fashion (approximating the neotongue), and the measurement is increased by 10%. The length is estimated by measuring from the base of tongue/larynx to the anterior mandible. The length is intentionally overestimated with plans to trim the excess distally during the flap inset. The flap is harvested with significant vastus lateralis muscle bulk, which sits in the submental area to help support the flap. The fascia of the vastus is used later to create a mandibular sling.

The flap is first inset posteriorly with an interrupted horizontal mattress technique and secured to the tongue base/pharynx or larynx. The flap is oriented with the pedicle directly posteriorly to either side of the neck. Interdental sutures are used along the remaining dentition as the inset is continued anteriorly. Interdental sutures, or suturing directly to the alveolar ridge, is preferred to sewing to the floor of mouth mucosa unless there is significant tissue that can be preserved. At the anterior portion of our reconstruction, the flap is trimmed in a fashion to create a conical pyramid that extends upward toward the hard palate (**Fig. 5**). This flap

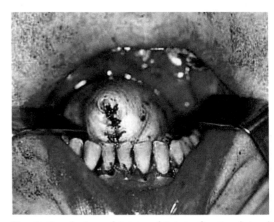

Fig. 5. Conclusion of intraoral inset of anterolateral thigh free flap for total glossectomy reconstruction.

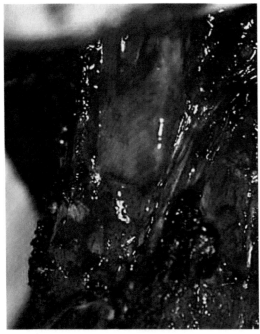

Fig. 4. Total glossectomy defect.

is secured with interdental sutures or sewn directly to the alveolar ridge mucosa in edentulous patients.

Suspension techniques are then performed in order to avoid the sinking of the flap with time. A mandibular sling is created by sewing the fascia of the vastus lateralis directly to small holes drilled through the inferior border of the mandible at 2-cm intervals from angle to angle (**Fig. 6**). Alternatively, a separate sling can be created by harvesting tensor fascia lata and securing this to the mandible to support the bulk of the flap in the submental area. In addition, a hyoid suspension is performed using large nonabsorbable sutures (**Fig. 7**). Two to 3 sutures around the hyoid bone are secured to the anterior mandible through the drill holes. This maneuver pulls the larynx superiorly and anteriorly to create bulk over the supraglottic base of the tongue area to reduce aspiration. Ten months after the reconstruction, the tongue still has adequate bulk and the patient can swallow without a gastrostomy tube (**Fig. 8**). **Table 1** provides a summary of recommendations.

LESSONS LEARNED IN TOTAL LARYNGOPHARYNGECTOMY RECONSTRUCTION

The total laryngopharyngectomy defect is particularly challenging, because it is prone to unfavorable functional results, most commonly caused by pharyngocutaneous fistulae and/or distal anastomotic stricture. Whether to reconstruct the defect with a tubed fasciocutaneous free flap or with an enteric jejunum flap has been a source of controversy in the literature for several decades. Anecdotally, the trend seems to have shifted toward the use of the fasciocutaneous flap reconstruction rather than the jejunum. This choice may be related

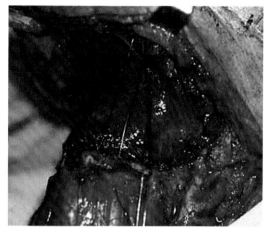

Fig. 7. A hyoid suspension is performed by securing the hyoid to mandible with 2.0 Prolene suture.

to the inherent morbidity of an open abdominal operation and to several investigators' concerns about so-called wet speech with jejunal flaps. Initial voice studies showed equivalent tracheoesophageal prosthesis (TEP) voice outcomes with radial forearm free flap reconstruction versus primary closure.[25] Subsequently, equivalent voice outcomes between radial forearm free flap versus anterolateral thigh free flap reconstruction have also been reported.[26]

Deschler and colleagues[27] compared tracheoesophageal voice quality in patients in 3 groups: primary closure, radial forearm free flap, and jejunal free flap reconstruction. This 2015 study compared novice and expert assessments of voice quality and the general quality-of-life outcomes measurements. The results showed inferior voice quality in all free flap patients (relative to primary closure) by both objective acoustic and subjective analyses. However, among the patients reconstructed with either type of free flap, voice outcomes were similar and voice-related

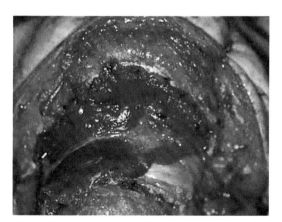

Fig. 6. Fascia is secured to holes drilled in the mandible to suspend flap.

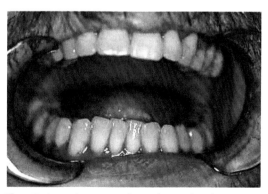

Fig. 8. Long-term results of total glossectomy reconstruction.

Table 1
Steps for avoiding unfavorable outcomes following total glossectomy reconstruction

Unfavorable Outcome	Steps to Limit Unfavorable Outcome
Atrophy of neotongue with loss of bulk	Choose a flap with significant adipose tissue: anterolateral thigh flap
Sagging of the neotongue	Suspend fascia of flap directly to drill holes in the mandible
Aspiration	Hyoid suspension helps prevent funneling of secretions
Dysarthria/dysphagia	Overestimate bulk of neotongue so that it makes contact with hard palate

quality-of-life measures were equivalent between all groups.[27]

Although it offers the optimal chance at TEP voice quality, performing primary closure of significant resection defects often results in stenosis. In addition, use of vascularized tissue may prevent the incidence and length of fistula, particularly in irradiated patients. This possibility was also recently addressed by Tan and colleagues,[28] comparing the results of radial forearm, anterolateral thigh, and jejunal free flap following a total laryngopharyngectomy using both an esophagram and endoscopic examination. They showed decreased, but not statistically significant, rates of fistula for jejunal and ALT free flaps versus radial forearm free flap (RFFF) (30%, 33%, and 50%, respectively). However, the rate of stricture was statistically significantly lower for jejunal free flaps (0%) versus ALT (38%) or RFFF (57%).[28]

Functional swallowing outcomes, as judged by return to normal or a soft diet, have also been compared for fasciocutaneous flaps (ALT/RFFF) versus jejunal free flaps. It may be that, given the natural peristalsis, mucosal lining, and secretory surface, the jejunal free flap would show improved swallowing outcomes in clinical studies. However, not all the published data supported this conclusion. A recent comparison of ALT, RFFF, jejunum, and supercharged jejunum showed a 96% return of swallowing with supercharged jejunum, 84% with RFFF, 69% with ALT, and only 67% with jejunum.[29] Several other studies have shown conflicting data as to the stricture rate and swallowing function following jejunal versus tubed cutaneous reconstruction.

Acknowledging the diverse published outcomes data, the practice at the UW has evolved over the past 20-plus years to preferentially use jejunal free flaps to reconstruct the total laryngopharyngectomy or cervical esophagectomy defects. The use of the enteric flap has, in our patients, resulted in better swallowing outcomes and lower stricture rates. Although the postoperative TEP speech outcomes are admittedly deeper and wetter, the postoperative fistula and stricture rates are lower in our procedures.

Surgical Tenets for Jejunal Free Flap Reconstruction

Key points to the selection, elevation, and inset of jejunal flaps at the UW are as follows:

- The jejunal free flap is only used when total cervical pharyngoesophagectomy defects are anticipated. For patients in whom even a 1-cm to 2-cm segment of the posterior (native) esophagus can be maintained, a 270° fasciocutaneous flap is used instead.
- Cooperation with an efficient general surgery team provides the selection of optimal arcade and harvest of a 12-cm to 15-cm segment of jejunum laparoscopically through a small (3–4 cm) incision in approximately an hour.
- Maintain isoperistaltic direction during inset (which is performed before vessel anastomosis).
- Inset jejunum with a small amount of stretch (it will subsequently elongate).
- Ensure 2-layer closure proximally and distally.
- Spatulate distal-end pharyngoesophageal border to minimize risk of stricture.
- A distal segment with 2 vascular arcades is subsequently externalized and used for a monitor segment (multiple arcades limit the risk of rotation and strangulation of the vascular supply).

Patient Presentation: Reconstruction of the Total Cervical Esophagectomy Defect

A 61-year-old man with a history of advanced laryngeal squamous cell carcinoma after total laryngectomy and postoperative radiotherapy 10 years before presentation. He returns with dysphagia and a neck mass found to be a new hypopharyngeal carcinoma (**Fig. 9**). Cross-sectional imaging confirmed dermal and circumferential involvement of the residual esophagus (**Fig. 10**) requiring a total cervical pharyngoesophagectomy (**Fig. 11**). An 8-cm segment of jejunum was harvested to replace the defect (**Fig. 12**) and an inset (**Fig. 13**) with a distal monitor

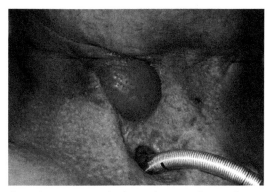

Fig. 9. Suprastomal hypopharyngeal carcinoma recurrence.

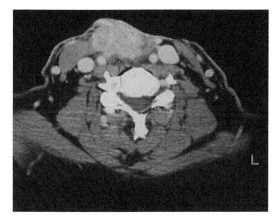

Fig. 10. Axial computed tomography scan showing recurrent hypopharyngeal cancer (*arrow*).

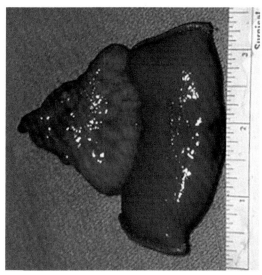

Fig. 12. Jejunal free flap following harvest.

paddle on 2 vascular arcades was mobilized through a skin incision (**Fig. 14**). To reconstruct the anterior skin and soft tissue defect, a pectoralis flap was elevated, inset, and covered with a split-thickness skin graft (**Fig. 15**). The 12-month post-operation appearance shows an acceptable cosmetic outcome, without evidence of strictures or recurrence (**Fig. 16**). **Table 2** provides a summary of recommendations.

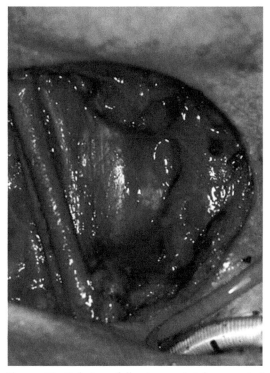

Fig. 11. Defect following total cervical pharyngoesophagectomy.

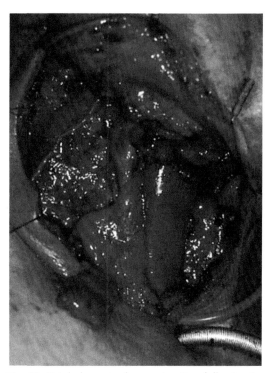

Fig. 13. Total pharyngeal reconstruction following jejunal flap.

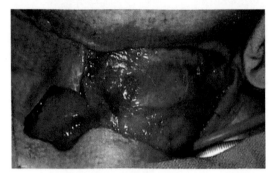

Fig. 14. Jejunal monitoring paddle.

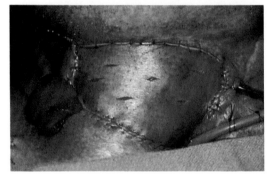

Fig. 15. Anterior cervical skin defect reconstructed with pectoralis flap and split-thickness skin graft.

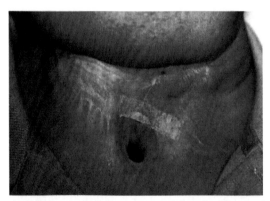

Fig. 16. One year following jejunal free flap for total pharyngectomy defect.

SUMMARY

Clinicians at UW have gained significant experience with head and neck free tissue transfers over the past 2 decades and, like most, continue to learn lessons from each reconstruction. This article presents 3 areas that the authors find particularly problematic when performing free tissue transfer to the head and neck. In terms of postoperative care, the authors recommend judicious use

Table 2
Steps for avoiding unfavorable outcomes during total laryngopharyngectomy reconstruction

Unfavorable Outcome	Steps to Limit Unfavorable Outcome
Dysphagia	Mucosally lined jejunal free flap results in better postoperative swallowing anecdotally
Wet tracheoesophageal speech	Fasciocutaneous flaps result in superior tracheoesophageal speech anecdotally
Distal pharyngeal stenosis	Spatulization of the proximal esophagus reduces anastomotic stenosis
Pharyngocutaneous fistula	Double-layered closure of jejunal anastomosis reduces risk of anastomotic leak

of tracheostomy tubes, liberal use of postoperative antibiotics (based on our recent published study), and the use of the traditional method for free flap monitoring, which involves frequent clinical examinations and pinprick testing.

For a total glossectomy defect, we recommend the use of the anterolateral thigh free flap with special attention to suspending the flap and larynx to the anterior mandible. For total laryngopharyngectomy defect, we recommend use of the jejunal enteric free flap. In addition, we support the notion of learning from each of our unfavorable results so that our subsequent patients may have even better outcomes.

REFERENCES

1. Hammerlid E, Mercke C, Sullivan M, et al. A prospective quality of life study of patients with oral or pharyngeal carcinoma treated with external beam irradiation with or without brachytherapy. Oral Oncol 1997;33(3):189–96.

2. Paula JM, Sonobe HM, Nicolussi AC, et al. Symptoms of depression in patients with cancer of the head and neck undergoing radiotherapy treatment: a prospective study. Rev Lat Am Enfermagem 2012;20(2):362–8.

3. Hammerlid E, Ahlner-Elmqvist M, Bjordal K, et al. A prospective multicentre study in Sweden and Norway of mental distress and psychiatric morbidity in head and neck cancer patients. Br J Cancer 1999; 80(5–6):766–74.

4. Hammerlid E, Silander E, Hörnestam L, et al. Health-related quality of life three years after diagnosis of head and neck cancer: a longitudinal study. Head Neck 2001;23(2):113–25.

5. Lydiatt WM, Bessette D, Schmid KK, et al. Prevention of depression with escitalopram in patients undergoing treatment for head and neck cancer: randomized, double-blind, placebo-controlled clinical trial. JAMA Otolaryngol Head Neck Surg 2013; 139(7):678–86.

6. Chew JY, Cantrell RW. Tracheostomy: complications and their management. Arch Otolaryngol 1972; 96(6):538–45.

7. Rao MK, Reilley TE, Schuller DE, et al. Analysis of risk factors for postoperative pulmonary complications in head and neck surgery. Laryngoscope 1992;102(1):45–7.

8. Coyle MJ, Tyrrell R, Godden A, et al. Replacing tracheostomy with overnight intubation to manage the airway in head and neck oncology patients: towards an improved recovery. Br J Oral Maxillofac Surg 2013;51(6):493–6.

9. Moore MG, Bhrany AD, Francis DO, et al. Use of nasotracheal intubation in patients receiving oral cavity free flap reconstruction. Head Neck 2010;32(8): 1056–61.

10. Moubayed SP, Barker DA, Razfar A, et al. Microvascular reconstruction of segmental mandibular defects without tracheostomy. Otolaryngol Head Neck Surg 2015;152(2):250–4.

11. Yarlagadda BB, Deschler DG, Rich DL, et al. Head and neck free flap surgical site infections in the era of the surgical care improvement project. Head Neck 2016;38(Suppl 1):E392–8.

12. Johnson JT, Myers EN, Thearle PB, et al. Antimicrobial prophylaxis for contaminated head and neck surgery. Laryngoscope 1984;94: 46–51.

13. Koshkareva YA, Johnson JT. What is the perioperative antibiotic prophylaxis in adult oncologic head and neck surgery? Laryngoscope 2014;124(5): 1055–6.

14. Bratzler DW, Dellinger EP, Olsen KM, et al. American Society of Health-System Pharmacists (ASHP); Infectious Diseases Society of America (IDSA); Surgical Infection Society (SIS); Society for Healthcare Epidemiology of America (SHEA). Clinical practice guidelines for antimicrobial prophylaxis in surgery. Surg Infect (Larchmt) 2013; 14(1):73–156.

15. Mitchell RM, Mendez E, Schmitt NC, et al. Antibiotic prophylaxis in patients undergoing head and neck free flap reconstruction. JAMA Otolaryngol Head Neck Surg 2015;141(12): 1096–103.

16. Khariwala SS, Le B, Pierce BH, et al. Antibiotic use after free tissue reconstruction of head and neck defects: short course vs. long course. Surg Infect (Larchmt) 2016;17(1):100–5.

17. Chae MP, Rozen WM, Whitaker IS, et al. Current evidence for postoperative monitoring of microvascular free flaps: a systematic review. Ann Plast Surg 2015;74(5):621–32.

18. May JW Jr, Chait LA, O'Brien BM, et al. The no-reflow phenomenon in experimental free flaps. Plast Reconstr Surg 1978;61(2):256–67.

19. Schmulder A, Gur E, Zaretski A. Eight-year experience of the Cook-Swartz Doppler in free-flap operations: microsurgical and reexploration results with regard to a wide spectrum of surgeries. Microsurgery 2011;31(1):1–6.

20. Weber RS, Ohlms L, Bowman J, et al. Functional results after total or near total glossectomy with laryngeal preservation. Arch Otolaryngol Head Neck Surg 1991;117(5):512–5.

21. Yun IS, Lee DW, Lee WJ, et al. Correlation of neotongue volume changes with functional outcomes after long-term follow-up of total glossectomy. J Craniofac Surg 2010;21(1):111–6.

22. Urken ML, Moscoso JF, Lawson W, et al. A systematic approach to functional reconstruction of the oral cavity following partial and total glossectomy. Arch Otolaryngol Head Neck Surg 1994; 120(6):589–601.

23. Effron MZ, Johnson JT, Myers EN, et al. Advanced carcinoma of the tongue: management by total glossectomy without laryngectomy. Arch Otolaryngol 1981;107(11):694–7.

24. Ruhl CM, Gleich LL, Gluckman JL. Survival, function, and quality of life after total glossectomy. Laryngoscope 1997;107(10):1316–21.

25. Alam DS, Vivek PP, Kmiecik J. Comparison of voice outcomes after radial forearm free flap reconstruction versus primary closure after laryngectomy. Otolaryngol Head Neck Surg 2008;139(2): 240–4.

26. Revenaugh PC, Knott PD, Alam DS, et al. Voice outcomes following reconstruction of laryngopharyngectomy defects using the radial forearm free flap and the anterolateral thigh free flap. Laryngoscope 2014;124(2):397–400.

27. Deschler DG, Herr MW, Kmiecik JR, et al. Tracheoesophageal voice after total laryngopharyngectomy reconstruction: Jejunum versus radial forearm free flap. Laryngoscope 2015;125(12): 2715–21.

28. Tan NC, Lin PY, Kuo PJ, et al. An objective comparison regarding rate of fistula and stricture among anterolateral thigh, radial forearm, and jejunal free tissue transfers in circumferential pharyngo-esophageal reconstruction. Microsurgery 2015;35(5):345–9.

29. Selber JC, Xue A, Liu J, et al. Pharyngoesophageal reconstruction outcomes following 349 cases. J Reconstr Microsurg 2014;30(9):641–54.

Henri Mondor Experience with Microsurgical Head and Neck Reconstruction Failure

Romain Bosc, MD*, Jean-Paul Meningaud, MD, PhD*

KEYWORDS

- Reconstructive surgery • Free flaps • Head and neck surgery • Mucosal reconstruction
- Dental rehabilitation • 3D planning

KEY POINTS

- The failure of a head and neck reconstruction even after a successful free flap transfer may be life-threatening if a drop in vital function is not restored.
- Simple plastic surgery techniques such as fat or skin autograft and local flaps are used to resolve sometimes complex issues without the need for a new major surgery.
- Inert reconstruction tissues in the oral cavity may impair the ability to swallow and phonation.
- Using surgical cutting guides for osteotomy results in better outcomes when a complex reconstruction of the mandibular or maxillary bone is needed.
- Allograft transplantation allows treating complex multitissular defects without free flap transfer and results in enhanced functional rehabilitation.

INTRODUCTION

Head and neck reconstruction surgery largely relies on the use of free flap techniques. The emergence and diffusion of microsurgery in the 1970s have marked a major change in the approach of the maxillofacial reconstruction surgery. In particular, it is now possible to consider complex reconstructions with a real functional and aesthetic rehabilitation potential.

However, microsurgery is a very demanding field. The progress with respect to the instrumentation (microscope, microinstruments) does not compensate for the difficulty of the surgical procedures. The learning curve is long, and considerable experience is necessary to ensure a satisfactory success rate.

The reconstructive surgeon is frequently faced with very complex decisions: donor site, recipient site, function to be rehabilitated, tissues to be reconstructed. It is sometimes impossible to fulfill all the requirements because of difficulties related to patient condition: salvage surgery, extensive and complex deterioration involving multiple tissues, adjuvant therapies (radiotherapy), precarious vascular status.

Surgeons concur that a truly successful reconstruction involves restitution, on the one hand, of essential functions: eating, phonation, oral continence, and respiration, and, on the other hand, restoration of the most aesthetically pleasing anatomy possible, compatible with a normal social life.

An unsatisfactory conformation of the transferred flap or a defective healing in the mouth will lead to functional rehabilitation failure. Conversely, too large of a tissue transfer will alter the functioning of residual anatomic structures such as the tongue or soft palate.

Service de Chirurgie Plastique, Reconstructrice, Esthétique et Maxillofaciale, Henri Mondor Hospital, 51 Avenue du Marechal de Lattre de Tassigny, Créteil 94000, France
* Corresponding author.
E-mail addresses: romainbosc@gmail.com; jean-paul.meningaud@hmn.aphp.fr

Clin Plastic Surg 43 (2016) 695–706
http://dx.doi.org/10.1016/j.cps.2016.05.008

In this article, the surgical techniques are discussed that allow improving the functions and aesthetic aspect when a free flap reconstruction has been carried out but with an insufficient functional or aesthetic result.

Discussed are the techniques used to improve the essential functions of swallowing, phonation, salivary continence, and the final morphologic result.

STANDARD PRACTICE

At the Henri Mondor teaching hospital, the authors treat patients with multiple injuries, ballistic injuries, and malformations (neurofibromatosis) and perform reconstructions after cancer therapy. Microsurgery was introduced in the 1980s. The adoption of microsurgical techniques by plastic surgeons has been very rapid, in particular for hand surgery and facial reconstructive surgery.

The use of free flaps for breast reconstruction after cancer therapy was adopted later, in the 1990s. The main free flaps used for maxillofacial bone reconstruction were fibula osteocutaneous flaps.

Other osteocutaneous flaps have been used: chimeric scapulodorsal, iliac crest, chimeric antebrachial, prefabricated flaps. It should be noted that 25 years after the fibula flap was first used, it remains, for the authors, the preferred technique when it is necessary to perform extensive mandibular and maxillary reconstruction (**Table 1**).

WHAT IS A FREE FLAP RECONSTRUCTION FAILURE?

Consider that there is a failure of the reconstruction in 2 different situations:

- The microsurgical free transfer fails with partial or total necrosis of the flap (partial or total necrosis of the skin paddle, necrosis of a fibular bone segment). The anatomic structure or function is not restored either partially (**Fig. 1**A) or totally (**Fig. 1**B).

- The microsurgical free transfer is functional, but one or several anatomic structures have not been reconstructed because of lack of tissues or failure to achieve satisfactory conformation of the transferred flap.

HOW IS HEAD AND NECK RECONSTRUCTION FAILURE MANAGED DESPITE A FREE FLAP SUCCESS?

It is necessary to carry out a precise semiological analysis of the patient anatomic and functional features to choose the technique that is the most suitable for the reconstruction of the missing structures.

Five issues related to the alteration of the essential anatomic structures are of interest and correspond to the main complaints of patients after reconstruction even when the free tissue transfer has been successful:

- Oral feeding
- Phonation and articulation
- Salivary continence
- Morphology and motor function of the face
- Infections and exposures of the osteosynthesis material

WHAT ARE THE ANATOMIC AND FUNCTIONAL STRUCTURES THAT SHOULD BE RESTORED?

A. The main problem faced after a partial failure of reconstruction is that of oral feeding.

Indeed, chewing and swallowing functions are extremely complex to restore after cancer surgery, even when the tissue transfers have been successful. These functions require an anatomic and functional restoration and a long rehabilitation. When one or more of these functions are not restored, feeding is compromised:

- Mobile tongue
- Soft palate and upper jaw
- Tongue base

Table 1
Classification of osteocutaneous flap qualities according to the parameters required for oral reconstruction after buccopharyngectomy and maxillectomy, ranked from A to D

| Flap | Tissue Flap Composition | | | Donor Site Parameters | |
	Bone Length	Skin Paddle	Pedicle	Position	Morbidity
Fibula	A	C	B	A	A
Scapula	C	B	B	D	D
Antebrachial	D	A	A	C	C
Iliac crest	B	D	D	B	C

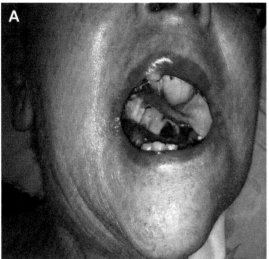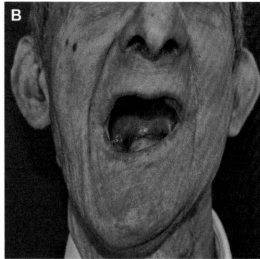

Fig. 1. (*A*) Reconstruction of the soft palate with a free antebrachial flap: total necrosis of the flap. (*B*) Partial necrosis of a fibular bone segment leading to mandibular deformity and dysfunction.

- Mandible
- Hypopharynx and oesophageal mouth

In addition, many patients undergo a gastrostomy or jejunostomy feeding tube before reconstruction surgery to help to maintain enteral feeding during the period when oral feeding is not possible.

In the authors' experience, the prolonged use of the enteral feeding tube leads to a progressive loss of neurologic and swallowing motor functions; this disturbs food resumption even when the anatomic structures have been successfully restored.

Finally, an additional problem sometimes occurs: when usually highly mobile structures such as the tongue or soft palate are reconstructed using inert tissues, including skin or muscle paddle, they may be a barrier to the route of the alimentary bolus.

Although it is possible to reconstruct a complete mobile tongue after total glossectomy with thigh anterolateral neurotized or deep inferior epigastric perforator (DIEP) flap, the authors think that it is preferable not to attempt to reconstruct the mobile tongue or mobile part of the soft palate when the patient is still able to be fed orally.

In the authors' experience, the recovery of neurotized flap sensitivity does not compensate for transferred tissue inertia and congestion, and this often results in a discomfort or complete blockage of liquid or solid food.

The decision to add additional reconstruction tissue is therefore based on a balance between the restoration needs of an organ and the risk of unbalancing the existing functions.

When a tongue reconstruction muscle or a fat flap disturbs oral feeding, the authors perform a defatting or partial resection guided by the clinical examination.

It is sometimes necessary to perform a second free or pedicled flap to restore the function or missing organ.

The choice of the flap depends, on the one hand, on the anatomic and functional structure to be restored (**Table 2**), and on the other hand, on the patient clinical status.

The pectoralis major musculocutaneous flap[1] and the latissimus dorsi musculocutaneus flap or the deltopectoral flap have disadvantages: scarring and lesions of the donor area (**Fig. 2**), and poor conformation of the skin paddle. However, they also have major advantages: rapid implementation, reliability of tissue transfer, and a large amount of tissue that may be transferred.

The techniques enable compensation for extensive mucosal tissue loss. The techniques are less primarily used; they are superseded by antebrachial flaps, because of the inferior functional results of the former.[2] Pedicled flaps are thus mainly used in salvage settings.   .

The facial artery musculomucosal (FAMM) flap and buccinator flap are of value in the partial reconstruction of the floor of the oral cavity,[3,4] while preserving lingual mobility (which is then generally left in controlled wound healing), but can only be used if the facial vessels have not been sacrificed for microsurgical anastomoses.

B. The second issue the authors face is the absence of a good salivary continence.

Table 2
Anatomic structure involved and preferred choice of reconstruction flap, ranked from A to E

	Fibula Flap	ALT Flap	Scapulodorsal Flap	Antebrachial Flap	Iliac Crest Flap
Mandibular bone	A	—	C	D	B
Tongue	C	A	D	B	E
Soft palate nasal floor	E	D	A	B	C
Alveolar ridge, buccal floor	C	B	D	A	E
Maxillary bone	C	—	B	—	A

Patients who have undergone a previous glossectomy extended to the vestibule, the lower lip, or the inner face of the cheek are reconstructed, most often using a fibula osteocutaneous free flap. Even when the reconstruction quality is very good, 2 issues may alter the result:

- Loss of sensitivity of the lower lip and vestibule related to the resection of one or both mandibular nerves[5]
- Insufficient depth of the anterior vestibule
- Insufficient height and motor function of the lower lip

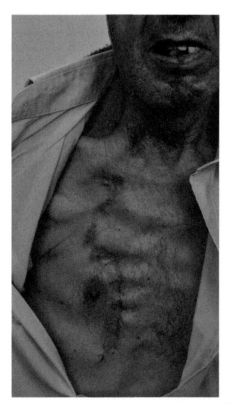

Fig. 2. Salvage surgery using a pectoralis major flap following necrosis of the skin paddle of a fibula osteocutaneous flap. Scarring sequelae.

These may result in a continual drooling, which seriously disables the patient, in particular for liquid absorption. Paradoxically, these symptoms may be less common in patients who have undergone radiotherapy due to the resulting oligoptyalism.

When this phenomenon occurs, it is necessary to carry out a deepening of the vestibule. If the facial artery has not been sacrificed by an ipsilateral lymph node resection and if the patient has not been irradiated, the authors primarily perform an FAMM mucosal flap.[4] To deepen the vestibule most often, they perform total skin grafts whose interposition is fixed with a bolster in the mouth (removed after 3 or 4 days). Total skin grafts in an "aesthetic unit" may also be used to increase the height of the lower lip and improve oral continence. Finally, they also use regularly the botulinum toxin to reduce saliva secretion.

C. The third problem the authors often face after free flap reconstruction is the modification or the inability to articulate properly.

Phonation is a complex function. Apart from the larynx, all structures of the oropharyngeal cavity are involved and each patient uses these mobile and fixed structures differently to talk:

- Oropharynx and hypopharynx
- Nasal floor and nasal cavities
- Soft palate
- Tongue and tongue base
- Lips
- Mandible

Modifying only one of these structures is sufficient to change the articulation. Usually, phonation remains completely possible (except in case of total laryngectomy) and rehabilitation sessions help patients to compensate for a defective functional structure. However, an incomplete or defective reconstruction of several anatomic structures may impair patient phonation, articulation, and understandability. For the same reasons as for feeding, an inert and voluminous tissue structure that blocks the inspiratory and expiratory air flow or impairs the residual mobility of the oropharynx will lead to dysarthria.

There are no specific surgical guidelines to restore a correct articulation and phonation. The main treatment is rehabilitation through physiotherapy and speech therapy. Nasality issues are treated, where possible, by performing soft palate or soft palate abutment plasty to improve their mobility. Total or subtotal palatal incompetencies are prevented by performing thin perforator flap reconstructions (fibula flap with lateral soleus perforator skin paddle). The authors also treat mandibular ankylosis and limited mouth opening with physiotherapy and botulinum toxin. In their experience, condylar surgery does not provide good results.

D. The morphologic aspect of the middle and lower third of the face may be greatly impaired after free flap reconstruction.

There are often marked differences in skin color on the paddles taken from the back, chest, or limbs. This difference in skin color results in a "patch" effect, which may decrease the final aesthetic score. Similarly, the presence of a hair area or area overloaded in fatty tissues on the chin or cheek is often poorly tolerated, in particular in women.

Facial paralysis after section of the facial nerve trunk or its branches leads to a static and dynamic facial deformity of variable severity, which should be corrected.

Relief or symmetry anomalies of the mandible reconstructed after transmaxillary buccopharyngectomy and fibula free flap are also often a cause of secondary corrective surgery. Finally, the poor bone restitution of the mandibular arch or teeth alters the final aesthetic score, possibly causing a major injury and a disability and preventing the return to a normal social life even when healing is achieved.

Through extension of the techniques applied to burn sequelae, the authors perform combined resurfacing associating deep dermabrasion, keratinocyte autografts (Recell), and lipofilling using a fine cannula. Trismus and facial paralysis sequella are treated with physiotherapy and botulinum toxin.

E. Finally, exposures of osteosynthesis material are common after fibula free flap reconstruction. They have several origins: infection, septic pseudoarthrosis and delayed consolidation of the fibula, intolerance to the osteosynthesis material, radiodermatitis, and scarring disunity of the skin paddle.

Treatment is mainly based on removal of exposed plates and screws. In most cases, the problem may be resolved.

Several preventive actions are useful to reduce this risk.

- The authors no longer use reconstruction macroplaques, which are less tolerated than screwed microplates.
- For fibula flap reconstructions, the authors try to only use bone segments longer than 2 cm. For shorter segments, the risk of osteonecrosis is increased (adventitious periostal stripping during modeling or osteosynthesis).
- The suture of the skin paddle in the mouth is made with extreme caution, with verification of the final impermeability and systematic resection of less vascularized areas.
- Intraoperative broad-spectrum antibiotic prophylaxis with penicillin A and clavulanic acid are used to decrease contamination and biofilm formation on the material.

HIGHLIGHT OF 2 UNFAVORABLE OUTCOMES UNRELATED TO FLAP NECROSIS AND HOW TO MANAGE THEM
Case 1

The case is presented of a patient who required an anterior glossectomy extended to the mandibular symphysis with fibula free flap reconstruction.

This 50-year old alcoholic patient who smoked (**Fig. 3**A) presented a large tumor with significant bicortical bone invasion (**Fig. 3**B). The local and regional extension assessment showed no synchronous tumor or remote metastasis.

Bone synthesis was carried out without difficulty from the deformable phantom of the native mandible (**Fig. 4**A). A single osteotomy was necessary for the modeling. Bone synthesis was carried out using screwed microplates. Mucosa reconstruction was performed using a simple skin paddle (**Fig. 4**B).

The initial reconstruction seemed satisfactory, but the healing process was marked by skin retractions deforming the lower lip. In addition, during radiotherapy, the patient presented a significant chin radiodermatitis and then skin ulceration, exposing the symphyseal osteosynthesis material (**Fig. 5**).

Local care and dressings led to the final healing.

Less than 2 years after the first surgery, the patient presented a suspicious vestibular ulceration on the resection edge. The biopsy confirmed squamous cell carcinoma recurrence.

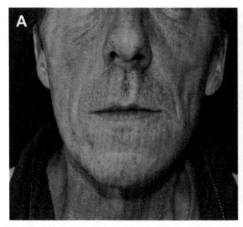
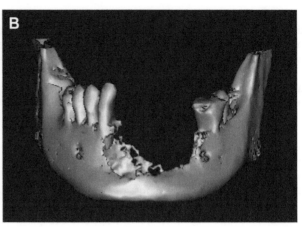

Fig. 3. (*A*) Squamous cell carcinoma of the buccal floor extended to the mandibular bone. (*B*) 3D volume rendering of the mandibular bone.

A new transfixing resection extending to the chin and including the previous reconstruction (**Fig. 6**A) was proposed with osteocutaneous chimeric antebrachial double skin paddle free flap reconstruction (**Fig. 6**B). The intraoperative result seemed satisfactory (**Fig. 6**C).

The histologic result showed a complete resection of the tumor recurrence in healthy margin. However, despite a good vascularization of the flap, the healing process was catastrophic with the following:

- A major ankyloglossia due to the retraction of the oral skin paddle
- A disappearance of the anterior vestibule
- A chin skin retraction on the bone fragments (**Fig. 7**)
- The disappearance of the chin projection

To improve the final result of this patient, the authors performed the following:

- A lower lip plasty to restore the continuity of the red lip with bilateral commissuroplasty
- A total intraoral skin graft to release ankyloglossia
- A complete symphyseal reconstruction with a new fibula flap with 2 skin paddles:
  - A perforating musculocutaneous paddle lifting on the lateral soleus vessels for the chin skin reconstruction in an "aesthetic unit"
  - A septocutaneous paddle for the reconstruction of the vestibule, alveolar ridge, and mouth floor

Case 2

The case is presented of a 55-year-old patient who underwent transmaxillary buccopharyngectomy

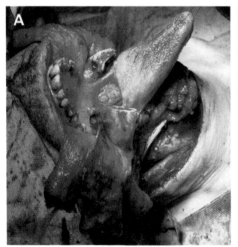
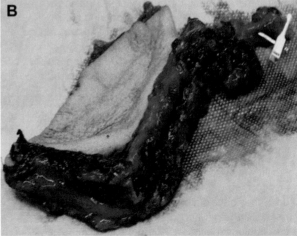

Fig. 4. (*A*) Interrupted anterior glossectomy extending to the ventral side of the tongue. (*B*) Intraoperative view of the fibula flap after modeling.

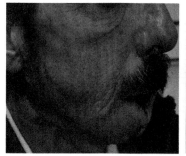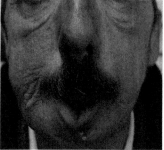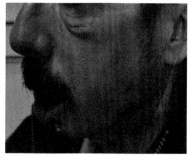

Fig. 5. Front, profile, and three-quarters views. V-shaped deformation of the lower lip. Insufficient lower lip height. Insufficient depth of the anterior vestibule. Chin skin ulceration and exposure of the osteosynthesis material.

with osteocutaneous fibula free flap reconstruction for squamous cell carcinoma of the right amygdala.

No difficulty occurred during surgery. The authors used a preformed titanium reconstruction plate.

After adjuvant treatment with radiotherapy, the patient presented an exposure of the osteosynthesis material on the chin and a hollowlike fibrous scar at the tragus area and right cheek (**Fig. 8**).

The tragus and cheek hollow were treated with 2 lipofilling sessions with a 2-month interval associated with a conventional cervicofacial lifting. The reconstruction titanium plate was removed during the same surgery. The outcome 1 year after the last surgery was considered very satisfactory by the patient (**Fig. 9**).

HOW CAN THE RELIABILITY OF OSTEOCUTANEOUS FREE FLAP RECONSTRUCTION BE ENHANCED?

Osteocutaneous flap reconstruction of the mandible or maxilla is a reliable and reproducible, but difficult to achieve, technique.

Several problems may occur and lead to a partial or total failure of the reconstruction even when the flap has been successful:

- Imperfect modeling with offset and poor dental articulation
- Necrosis or partial lysis of an osteotomy fragment
- Delayed healing/pseudoarthrosis leading to a deformation

All these complications may require further surgeries for improvement.

The authors prefer to leave a latency period of at least 6 to 12 months between the end of radiotherapy and the start of rehabilitation procedures.

They first perform a complete clinical examination to rule out a local cancer recurrence, uncontrolled infectious or inflammatory process: septic pseudoarthrosis, osteonecrosis, and exposure of the osteosynthesis material. They evaluate reconstruction stiffness, joint movement amplitudes and the mouth opening.

A head and neck computed tomography (CT) angiography is used to assess the quality of

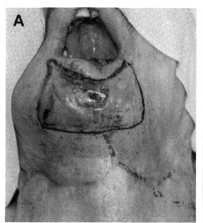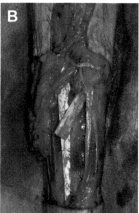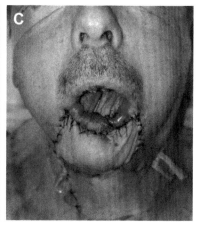

Fig. 6. (*A*) Symphyseal transfixing resection extended to the ventral side of the mobile tongue, chin, and white lip. (*B*) Osteocutaneous chimeric antebrachial double skin paddle flap. (*C*) Immediate postoperative result.

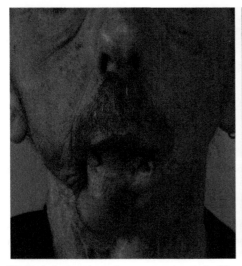
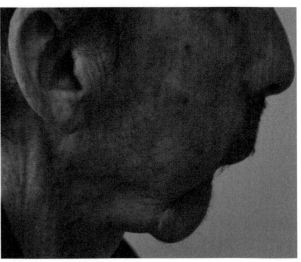

Fig. 7. Anterior glossectomy reconstructed with an osteocutaneous chimeric antebrachial double skin paddle free flap.

reconstructed bone structures. Volume- and surface-rendering images are used to determine the exact areas of concern: insufficient or excessive length of a bone segment, problem of symphyseal, or ramus angulation.

Bone lengths less than 2 cm are managed by interposing an iliac or tricortical scapular graft.

The major improvement that the authors have implemented for 3 years is the use of a total planning of the reconstruction surgery and the production of customized cutting guides through rapid prototyping.

The principle is to use volume-rendering and surface-rendering records produced from the patient CT angiography to design, by computer-aided design (CAD), the authors' own guides and titanium plates.

They evaluated the feasibility of producing their own cutting guides without the intervention of an

outside laboratory for patients with cancer undergoing mandibulectomy.

For 3 years, the authors have been producing their own customized cutting guides using computer-assisted design techniques and 3-dimensional (3D) printing.

The guides greatly facilitate mandibular and fibular osteotomies even for surgeons with relatively little experience of the procedures (**Fig. 10**).

The customized cutting guides may be combined with titanium plates that have been conformed and cut to measure using 3D printed reconstruction models (**Fig. 11**).

Reconstructing quality improvement after a free transfer failure is more important. In particular, the 3D planning helps to choose the optimal conformation of the fibula and provides osteosynthesis

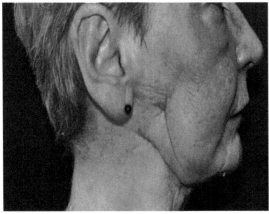
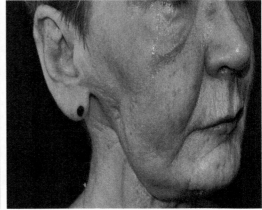

Fig. 8. Three-quarters and right profile views. Postoperative view, 1 year after right transmaxillary buccopharyngectomy.

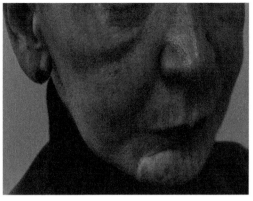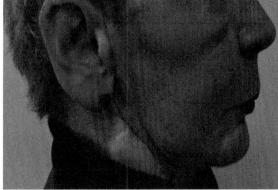

Fig. 9. Three-quarters and profile views: treatment with 2 sessions of fat autograft + cervicofacial lifting.

lines more suitable for the mandibular mechanics: step-osteotomies.

Visualizing the peroneal vessels, neck vessels, musculocutaneous and septocutaneous perforators allows optimizing the osteotomy lines to reduce the risk of lesion of the vascularization or skin paddles and prepare bone segments long enough to ensure the sustainability of their vascularization (**Fig. 12**).

The planning tools are also used to provide a reconstruction mode taking into account the previous surgeries. When osteosyntheses have already been carried out and show no difficulty, the planning will enable using the material already in place to optimize the operating time and avoid repeating the entire reconstruction.

IN CASE OF NEED FOR A NEW FREE FLAP, HOW SHOULD THE RECIPIENT VASCULAR SITE BE EVALUATED?

Reconstructions are implemented by tissue transfer. After an initial free flap use, the quality of the recipient site should be rigorously evaluated, particularly the presence of veins and arteries of sufficient caliber suitable for anastomosis. If the branches of the external carotid artery were consumed or ligated during the first procedure, it is necessary to check whether a sufficiently long and patent adequate external carotid artery stump remains.

It is possible to create a venous end-to-side anastomosis to the internal jugular vein. The authors do not perform microvascular anastomoses to the internal or common carotid artery. In the authors' experience, clamping the internal carotid in that context has a high potential for morbidity (embolism, stroke, secondary thrombosis, carotid dissection).

The authors prefer anastomosis to the external carotid artery rather than to one of its branches (facial, thyroid, or pharyngeal artery) to ensure a more favorable arterial blood flow.

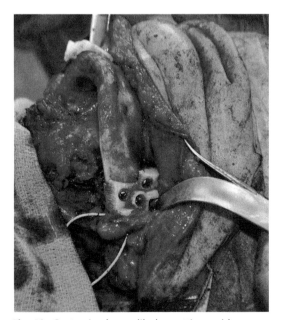

Fig. 10. Customized mandibular cutting guides.

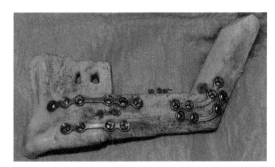

Fig. 11. Titanium mesh plate shaping on 3D printed model fibular reconstruction.

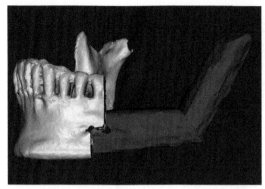

Fig. 12. Model of fibula reconstruction with step-osteotomies.

The use of 3D reconstruction software, with volume rendering, enables imaging of the vasculature of the neck and planning the anastomosis sites.

If the vasculature of the reconstruction side is not satisfactory, contralateral vessel bypass is possible with saphenous vein graft.

WHICH FLAP SHOULD BE SELECTED?

In the anterolateral thigh (ALT) flap, the tissue volume is greater than that with an antebrachial flap, whereas its fasciocutaneous composition ensures stability after radiotherapy.[6,7]

The choice between an antebrachial and ALT flap is governed not only by the magnitude of the

tissue loss but also by patient morphology. In obese patients, the indications for an antebrachial flap are extended to include tissue loss exceeding half a mobile tongue; for thin or malnourished patients, an ALT flap is preferable.

The authors also use an ALT flap when it is not possible to obtain an antebrachial flap or when the latter has already been removed from the nondominant arm; this prevents the risk of a lesion on the dominant forearm or hand.

The donor site sequelae are acceptable and considered by several investigators[6,7] to be less severe than those associated with antebrachial flap removal. In the event of failure of an initial ALT flap, it is possible to remove a flap from the contralateral thigh after having verified that perforators are present.

The antebrachial flap remains a valuable tissue donor site when isolated mucosal or cutaneous reconstruction is necessary. The amount of tissue available enables de-epidermization and reconstruction of several organs or functions:

- Mouth floor and mobile tongue
- Nasal fossae floor and palate

When necessary, the authors have used other flaps for head and neck omentum flap; DIEP flap; thoracodorsal artery perforator flap; chimeric free latissimus dorsi flap; free parascapular flap; contralateral fibula chimeric flap (**Table 3**).

Table 3
Choice of corrective techniques after free flap reconstruction failure (last 20 years)

Free Flap Success for Head and Neck Reconstruction	Number of Patient with at Least a Second Surgery Needed (%)	Technique Used for the Second Surgery	Number of Second Surgeries (%)
Fibula flap (46)	23 (50)	Skin graft Fibula flap Antebrachial flap Iliac crest graft Face transplant	9 (39.1) 7 (30.4) 2 (8.7) 1 (4.3) 4 (17.5)
ALT flap (13)	4 (30.7)	Skin graft Antebrachial flap ALT flap	2 (50) 1 (25) 1 (25)
Antebrachial flap (62)	14 (22.5)	Skin graft FAMM flap Latissimus dorsi flap ALT flap	7 (50) 4 (28.5) 2 (14.25) 1 (7.25)
Epiploic flap (5)	5 (100)	Skin graft Face transplant Skin graft Frontal pedicled flap	4 (80) 1 (20) 1 (33.3) 1 (33.3)

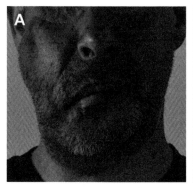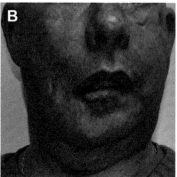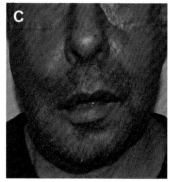

Fig. 13. Evolution of allograft over 5 years and after several corrective surgeries: (*A*) 6 months after the allograft: labial commissuroplasty. (*B*) Two years after the allograft: cutaneous resection of the chin and neck. (*C*) Four years after the allograft: cervical lifting and maxillar osteotomy.

HOW TO PROCEED WHEN THE TISSUE DEFECTS ARE TOO EXTENSIVE AND SEVERAL TISSUE TRANSFERS ARE NECESSARY? MULTITISSULAR ALLOGRAFT

In the authors' experience, reconstruction is rarely satisfactory in patients presenting with very extensive intermediate and inferior facial lesions, particularly in the event of complete destruction of the orbicular muscle of the mouth. The number of neurotized tissue transfers is too great and even neurotized muscle transfers do not enable the appearance and function of the lips to be restored. In such extreme cases, the authors used to propose a composite allograft. The advantage of the technique is that it provides a great deal of tissues and enables the functions of damaged organs to be restored. In the last 6 years, the authors have participated to 7 face allografts.[8,9]

Among the patients, 5 had previously had free flaps. There were 4 cases of ballistic injury; 1 patient was a burn victim.

One patient died after the graft, but all the other patients experienced an initial significant improvement in their reconstructions, in particular in the facial motor function and aesthetic aspect.

Patients may return to a better social and professional life.

However, several problems remain.

Despite adapted immunosuppressive therapy, some transplant patients experience a chronic rejection equivalent, which progressively impairs the graft: skin ulcers, discoloration, delayed bone consolidation, neuroma. Currently, patients grafted in France experienced subacute rejection episodes threatening the graft. Other patients with limb allografts (forearm) have experienced

the same problem, and graft removal was necessary.

- Several other problems have arisen in transplant patients:
  - The graft combining the upper and lower jaw has required complex corrective osteotomies to restore satisfactory bone continuity between the recipient and the graft (**Fig. 13**).
  - Airway issues related to the absence of sinus cavity graft have occurred.
  - The absence of hemifacial motor function in some patients due to an abnormal nerve anastomosis or incomplete nerve regrowth has occurred. Corrective commissuroplasties with the use of botulinum toxin have been needed.

The hindsight on these techniques is still insufficient to propose this treatment in routine care. Currently, in France, the technique is not proposed for patients presenting with surgical sequelae in a context of malignant tumor due to the risk of disease recurrence related to immunosuppressive treatment. However, some teams have suggested expanding the indications to include patients who have been in remission for more than 5 years.

SUMMARY

In the authors' practice, the use of new surgical assistance technologies, that is, cutting guides, virtualization of the stages of surgery, and 3D printing, have markedly reduced the reconstructive failures related to poor conformation of the osteocutaneous chimeric flaps used in maxillary and mandibular reconstruction. However, complex situations, related to the patient precarious vascular status or the extent of the tissues to be reconstructed, still occur.

Simple techniques such as skin or mucosa grafting, local mucosal flaps, and VY-shaped extension flaps, may improve tongue and soft palate mobility. These techniques may help to deepen the vestibule and correct lip continence.

The flaps, providing a significant tissue volume, may alter residual functions and should only be used sparingly.

Apart from reconstructions after cancer, composite tissue allograft is, in the authors' opinion, the only technique that enables reconstruction of the face when the lesions are very extensive and the orbicular muscle of the mouth has been totally destroyed. The authors' experience in the field of face transplants has led them to adopt a different approach to patients presenting with severe tissue defects after ballistic injury. They prefered to directly propose allograft rather than several free flaps with a non-negligible risk of failure associated with each procedure.

More than 10 years later, despite the significant hope raised by the first allografts of the face, the results are still mixed and insufficient.

REFERENCES

1. Milenovic A, Virag M, Uglesic V, et al. The pectoralis major flap in head and neck reconstruction: first 500 patients. J Craniomaxillofac Surg 2006;34:340–3.

2. Su WF, Hsia YJ, Chang YC, et al. Functional comparison after reconstruction with a radial forearm free flap or a pectoralis major flap for cancer of the tongue. Otolaryngol Head Neck Surg 2003; 128:412–8.

3. Ayad T, Kolb F, De Mones E, et al. The musculo-mucosal facial artery flap: harvesting technique and indications. Ann Chir Plast Esthet 2008;53:487–94 [in French].

4. Pribaz J, Stephens W, Crespo L, et al. A new intraoral flap: facial artery musculomucosal (FAMM) flap. Plast Reconstr Surg 1992;90:421–9.

5. Cordeiro PG, Schwartz M, Neves RI, et al. A comparison of donor and recipient site sensation in free tissue reconstruction of the oral cavity. Ann Plast Surg 1997;39:461–8.

6. Loreti A, Di Lella G, Vetrano S, et al. Thinned antero-lateral thigh cutaneous flap and radial fasciocutaneous forearm flap for reconstruction of oral defects: comparison of donor site morbidity. J Oral Maxillofac Surg 2008;66:1093–8.

7. Valentini V, Cassoni A, Marianetti TM, et al. Antero-lateral thigh flap for the reconstruction of head and neck defects: alternative or replacement of the radial forearm flap? J Craniofac Surg 2008;19: 1148–53.

8. Lantieri L, Hivelin M, Audard V, et al. Feasibility, reproducibility, risks and benefits of face transplantation: a prospective study of outcomes. Am J Transplant 2011;11:367–78.

9. Meningaud JP, Hivelin M, Benjoar MD, et al. The procurement of allotransplants for ballistic trauma: a preclinical study and a report of two clinical cases. Plast Reconstr Surg 2011;127:1892–900.

Liverpool Opinion on Unfavorable Results in Microsurgical Head and Neck Reconstruction: Lessons Learned

James Brown, MD, FRCS, FDSRCS[a,b,*], Andrew Schache, PhD, FRCS, FDSRCS[a,b], Chris Butterworth, MPhil, FDSRCS, FDS(Rest), RCS(Eng)[c,d]

KEYWORDS

- Reconstruction • Microsurgery • Microvascular • Flap transfer • Mandible • Maxilla
- Head and neck • Complications • Pitfalls

KEY POINTS

- Soft tissue reconstruction of the oral cavity.
  - Resect oncologically, aware that maintenance of the patient's own tissue, with a maintained blood and nerve supply, is ideal.
  - Excess tissue in partial tongue reconstruction can result in poorer function.
  - The remaining oral tongue must have optimum movement.
  - Extensive oral tongue resections require more bulk so that the swallow is initiated with little chance of effective chewing because the functioning tongue is more essential than an occluding dentition.
  - The floor of the mouth and buccal tissues require a thin flap to allow good movement.
  - Think of the oral tissues and soft palate as horizontal with less need of a sphincteric affect and the rest of the oropharynx as vertical where the sphincteric effect is paramount.
- Mandibular reconstruction.
  - Segmental resections involving the anterior mandible present more significant challenges than the posterior mandible, where a variety of techniques are used. The height of remaining bone in the anterior mandible and its relationship to the circumoral musculature is critical in the degree of postoperative collapse and the likelihood of effective rehabilitation.
- Maxillary reconstruction.
  - For low level defects (Brown class I and II), maxillary obturation is effective especially if supported by osseointegrated dental and zygomatic implants.
  - Zygomatic implants can be used in conjunction with soft tissue free flaps to effectively rehabilitate patients without the need for composite reconstruction with the associated technical complications and additional morbidity.
  - Maxillary defects involving the orbital floor (Class III) require composite free flaps to effect a satisfactory facial reconstruction and dental rehabilitation.
  - When the orbit is removed (Class IV) the facial profile can be managed with a prosthesis, but dental rehabilitation may still require a composite flap.
  - Collaboration with the team providing final rehabilitation and prosthetic support is essential before deciding on the reconstruction.

[a] Department of Head and Neck Surgery, Aintree University Hospital, Lower Lane, Liverpool L9 7AL, UK; [b] Northwest Cancer Research Centre, Liverpool University, London Road, Liverpool L39 9TA, UK; [c] Maxillofacial Prosthodontics, Aintree University Hospital, Lower Lane, Liverpool L9 7AL, UK; [d] Prosthodontic Department, Liverpool University Dental Hospital, Pembroke Place, Liverpool L3 5PS, UK
* Corresponding author. Department of Head and Neck Surgery, Aintree University Hospital, Lower Lane, Liverpool L9 7AL, UK.
E-mail address: brownjs@doctors.org.uk

Clin Plastic Surg 43 (2016) 707–718
http://dx.doi.org/10.1016/j.cps.2016.05.007
0094-1298/16/$ – see front matter © 2016 Elsevier Inc. All rights reserved.

INTRODUCTION

We have been given a title that asks the Liverpool head and neck reconstructive group for an opinion on "unfavorable" microsurgical reconstruction and asks "what lessons have been learned."[1–4] This is a personal view, although these opinions have been formed after much collaboration with the co-authors and also additional surgeons involved with the care of the patient, nurses, speech therapists, dietitians, and radiation oncologists. Good reconstruction, which is long-lasting and resilient, makes an enormous difference to a patient who may frequently have lost aesthetics and function through ablative cancer surgery. Although evidence to support this is found in the literature in the form of outcome questionnaire and assessments, the most valuable perspective is derived from the personal experiences gained in the outpatient clinic during the prolonged process of review for this patient group.

It is important to understand the difference between reconstruction for a patient following ablative head and neck cancer surgery and those that have suffered maxillofacial injuries. Trauma patients have no choice in the predicament they find themselves and hope that the reconstruction will improve their final result in a normal life span. A patient with cancer requires to be consented to undergo a potentially damaging procedure in terms of function and aesthetics and hence the reconstructive option and predicted outcome becomes part of the process of consent. Chemoradiotherapy, as an alternative to ablative surgery for organ preservation especially in the larynx and oropharynx, is well-recognized and hence the difference in outcome and function is paramount and still controversial to some extent. Laced in with this argument is also the impact on survival by withholding ablative surgery. Most of our experience has been with the patient with head and neck cancer and so it is with these patients in mind that this article is written.

In my time in surgery I have trained many individuals in complex ablation and reconstruction for the patient with head and neck cancer including the skull base. As a young surgeon starting off, it is essential to achieve free flap transfer success to gain the support of skeptical colleagues, but mostly to fulfill your planned treatment of the patient. This advice is not as good as a training position where one can follow the actions of accomplished surgeons in avoiding and then dealing with poor outcomes.

Potential comorbidities that may either influence the decision to avoid free flap reconstruction or, alternatively, inform a more appropriate flap choice from the ideal in the primary site (ultimate form, function, and rehabilitation) include

1. Previous bilateral neck surgery
2. Previous radiotherapy and especially chemoradiotherapy to the head and neck
3. Previous failed microvascular techniques
4. Peripheral vascular disease
5. Type II diabetes
6. Sickle cell disease or coagulopathy

In such circumstances the risk of failure may be such that the surgeon and the patient believe that the risks outweigh benefit.

In our practice we are always careful when advising a patient on a reconstructive option when a neck dissection and radiotherapy have already been performed. In such cases it is essential to carefully consider a simpler option than a free flap with the caveat that if unsatisfactory then complex reconstruction can still be considered. In general there is ample evidence in the literature to show that flap failure is not related to obesity or old age, although surgical complications in general may have a more damaging effect on the patient's recovery.

Even in the modern era of microvascular reconstructive surgery there are only a few flaps that are used regularly and fibula is by far the most common option for composite reconstruction of the mandible.[5] Any microvascular reconstruction requires considerable skill and surgeons with this training should be confident in most free tissue transfer techniques including iliac crest, scapula, and the incorporation of perforator flaps for both these donor sites.[6,7] The quality of the primary site reconstruction and overall result for the patient is paramount, so selection of the most appropriate reconstruction from the point of view of good rehabilitation is essential, aided by a comprehensive armamentarium of flap options. In Liverpool, the optimum reconstruction to provide the best outcome is selected if the patient is sufficiently medically fit and psychologically prepared to consent for the proposed procedure. Essential in the decision regarding composite tissue loss is the role of the maxillofacial prosthodontist with a special interest in the oral and facial rehabilitation for these patients.

COMMENT ON NONMICROVASCULAR RECONSTRUCTION FOR THE PATIENT WITH HEAD AND NECK CANCER

The most important decision for the patient typically via a tumor board (North America) or multidisciplinary team (United Kingdom) is the offer of ablative surgery as part of their cancer treatment.

There must be clarity as to whether this is a curative or a palliative option because the resection and reconstruction are complex and the sequellae long lasting. The role of microvascular reconstructive surgery is discussed later; however, it is essential that the surgeon be aware of, and carefully consider, local and pedicled flap options that may be more appropriate depending on the defect and the comorbidity of the patient. This form of surgery is useful in dealing with complications of microvascular reconstructions where dehiscence, fistula formation, or flap loss may have occurred. Readers are no doubt aware of the varied and useful flaps available in the head and neck and chest region (see later) but I emphasize the introduction of the supraclavicular artery island flap and the internal mammary perforator flap, both of which are used around the lower neck in particular, to treat or reinforce attempts to close oropharyngocutaneous fistulas or problems around tracheal stomas. These flaps are well-described by Fernandes.[8] Nonmicrovascular reconstructive flap options include the following:

1. Forehead
2. Nasolabial
3. Submental island
4. Temporoparietal fascia
5. Temporalis muscle
6. Pectoralis major
7. Latissimus dorsi
8. Sternocleidomastoid
9. Trapezius
10. Supraclavicular island
11. Internal mammary artery perforator

We still use the forehead and glabella flaps, temporalis, and especially the temporoparietal flap for augmentation and treatment of dehiscence following successful free tissue transfers for the maxillectomy defect. I have found that most patients, depending on their age and expectations, do not wish additional major surgery if a reasonable result can be achieved more quickly and simply (**Fig. 1**).

AVOIDING POOR RESULTS AFTER SUCCESSFUL FREE FLAP TRANSFER FOR SOFT TISSUE RECONSTRUCTION OF THE ORAL CAVITY AND OROPHARYNX
Oral Cavity

It is not possible to reconstruct the tongue either in the oral cavity (mobile or anterior tongue) or the oropharynx, where we refer to it as the posterior tongue. In our experience the functional results after three-quarter or total oral tongue resection are often less detrimental than the similar extent of resection for the posterior tongue. Primary surgery with or without postoperative radiotherapy remains the standard of care for squamous cell carcinoma of the oral cavity and it is fortunate that the reconstruction of the tongue (up to three-quarter partial glossectomy of the anterior tongue), floor of the mouth, retromolar region, the buccal mucosa, and the oral mucosa in general is reliable, particularly with respect to free tissue transfer techniques.

In our practice the radial forearm fasciocutaneous flap remains at the forefront of our decision-making when segmental resection of mandible is not necessary. The main argument against the

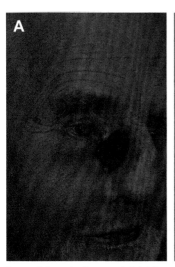
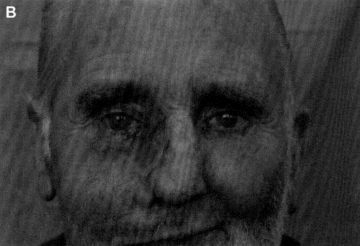

Fig. 1. (*A*) Typical potential dehiscence site for a patient reconstructed with a vascularized iliac crest with internal oblique following a maxillectomy (class IIId). (*B*) Defect treated with a silastic cover giving a good result for eye support and general appearance. The patient did not wish a biologic flap solution.

use of this flap is the donor site morbidity, because often a skin graft is required to close the donor site, although sensation to the hand and normal hand function are preserved with care during the harvest. Certainly the lower arm is not a site favored by patients[4] and slow healing of the grafted site can result in an ugly scar. There was a period when we used the lateral arm flap[9] because this could be closed directly and because it is sited above the elbow, the scar remains less obtrusive (**Fig. 2**), but the ability to raise the flap during the resection is more limited and most surgeons looking for a radial alternative now favor a perforator flap raised from the anterolateral thigh[10] or the lower limb.[11,12] The main advantage of the lateral arm or lower limb perforator options versus the anterolateral thigh flap is that these flaps are thin and pliable making them ideal for oral soft tissue contour reconstruction.

Oropharynx

In the oropharynx the tongue, although less mobile, plays a vital role in the initiation and completion of a successful swallow and contributes to effective protection of the vocal cords and trachea. Fortunately chemoradiotherapy has shown equivalent disease control levels as primary surgery with or without postoperative radiotherapy and so in our practice we rarely offer extensive posterior tongue resection as a primary treatment option, if a free flap reconstruction is required. However, we use transoral laser surgery to resect smaller tumors in the oropharynx, which does not require free tissue transfer maintaining the sphincteric effect of the surrounding musculature so vital to function. Transoral laser techniques were popularized by Steiner and coworkers,[13] but these techniques also work well in the oropharynx with good disease control and functional outcomes. Reconstruction of the pharyngeal walls and soft

palate is achieved and we have described the use of the superiorly based pharyngeal flap combined with a radial forearm flap, which we still use.[14] This allows healing and contracture to take place especially after postoperative radiotherapy and prevents anterior displacement of the flap away from the posterior pharyngeal wall with inevitable velopharyngeal incompetence. For most extensive oropharyngeal resections we previously used the rectus abdominus myocutaneous flap but now prefer the anterolateral thigh flap because this can easily be raised simultaneous to the resection and provides sufficient bulk to replace the posterior tongue allowing a safe swallow to be possible with potentially reduced donor site morbidity risk.

AVOIDING POOR RESULTS AFTER SUCCESSFUL FLAP TRANSFER FOR MANDIBULAR RECONSTRUCTION

In the microvascular reconstruction of the mandible the predominant donor sites are the fibula, iliac crest, scapula, and radial.[5] **Table 1** shows the flaps best suited to each defect of the mandible as recently classified.[5] In Liverpool we generally prefer the iliac crest to the fibula for dentate patients requiring a hemimandibulectomy (including the ipsilateral canine but not the condyle [class II]), and for the central defect [class III] to maintain adequate height to support the chin and implants. If the hemimandibulectomy requires a condylectomy (class IIc) then the fibula is easier to use given the increased bone length and reduced fullness in the condylar region. The fibula would also be our first choice for extensive mandibular defects in which both canines and at least one angle are resected (three corners of the mandible or more: class IV).[5]

There is a paucity of published data to support flap choice if the fibula is a compromised donor site, mainly as a result of peripheral vascular disease or occasionally an anatomic variant when the peroneal artery is the major blood supply to the foot. In the Liverpool region there is a high proportion of people from a lower socioeconomic base and a high level of smoking contributing to peripheral vascular disease in particular. We are in the process of publishing our experience with patients requiring mandibular resection for which a fibula is the preferred option but the magnetic resonance angiography that is performed for all these patients is unfavorable (C. Barry, et al, unpublished data, 2016). In this report we had 77 patients considered for a fibula but 20 (26%) of these had an unfavorable magnetic resonance angiography and were treated with scapula (eight cases), iliac crest (six cases), and radial forearm flaps (six

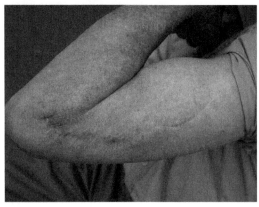

Fig. 2. The lateral arm donor site scar.

Table 1
Flap preference related to the length and type of mandibular defect

Class	Preference			
	Most Preferred	Second Best	Third Best	Least Preferred
I (Lateral: both angles but not ipsilateral canine or condyle)	Fibula, iliac crest, scapula equal merit			Radial
Ic (Lateral and condyle)	Fibula	Iliac crest and scapula equal merit		Radial
II (Anterolateral: Ipsilateral canine and both angles not condyle)	Iliac crest	Fibula	Scapula	Radial
IIc (Anterolateral and condyle)	Fibula and iliac crest equal merit		Scapula	Radial
III (Anterior: bilateral canines)	Iliac crest	Fibula	Scapula	Radial
IV (Extensive: bilateral canines and at least one angle)	Fibula	Iliac crest, scapula equal merit		Radial
IVc (Extensive and condyle(s))	Fibula	Radial	Iliac crest, scapula equal merit	

If soft tissue loss is a major issue then often the scapula donor site is preferred, either using the circumflex scapula and well-supplied skin or a latissimus dorsi perforator flap and scapula tip if pedicle length becomes a problem.

Data from Brown JS, Barry C, Ho MW, et al. A new classification for mandibular defects after oncological resection. Lancet Oncol 2016;17(1):e23–e30.

cases). In this collection of data over 5.5 years during the period 2008 to 2014 there were 172 osseous free flaps of which 77 were fibulas, 37 scapulas, 33 iliac crests, and 25 composite radials demonstrating our departmental philosophy of offering the full range of composite flaps, with the defect dictating the flap choice rather than vice versa. There seems to be little difference in flap survival when large series are reported between the flap options. In 150 consecutive osseous free flaps reported from Memorial Sloan-Kettering from 1999 onward there were 135 fibulas, six radials, six scapulas, and three iliac crest demonstrating the reliance on the fibula donor site, albeit all the flaps were successful.[15] During development of the recently published classification,[5] I reviewed 167 papers from 1990 to 2013 where more than 10 mandibular reconstructions were included, and can report the overall flap failure rates for those reported, of 128 of 3317 (3.9%) for fibula, 51 of 789 (6.5%) iliac crest, 20 of 481 (4.1%) radius, and 18 of 460 (3.8%) for scapula from 145 publications. This indicates a marginally higher failure rate for the iliac crest, which may be associated with the small caliber of the vessels and the technically more demanding harvest. These small differences mean little to patients during consent and there are many other reasons for failure apart from the chosen donor site depending on the case. From these data it is clear that the success of composite free tissue transfer in

mandibular reconstruction is generally a safe procedure with a low flap failure record. Compromising choice of flap to ensure flap survival is not supported by the high success rates for all routinely used composite free flaps.

It has been argued that the morbidity associated with some donor sites is unacceptable and especially in relation to the split radius and full-thickness iliac crest. The experience gained from using each of these flaps within our unit does not support this suggestion. Although not blinded to the flap type, an external orthopedic auditing of our practice[16] demonstrated similar outcomes for the patients irrespective of composite flap donor site. I have never regretted using the iliac crest and internal oblique donor site in head and neck reconstructive surgery. In Liverpool we still use the composite radial forearm flap even though we have reported a high donor site fracture rate of 17%,[17] but that predated evidence from Villaret and Futran,[18] which showed that prophylactic platting of the radius protected the patient from this debilitating fracture. The composite radial forearm flap remains useful to restore mandibular continuity but the bone, although well-vascularized, if raised from the ulnar side is thin and dental rehabilitation is compromised. This flap, however, is useful in edentulous (Cawood and Howell class V-VI) ridges,[19] especially if the fibula is not available and implant rehabilitation is not deemed to be important for the patient.

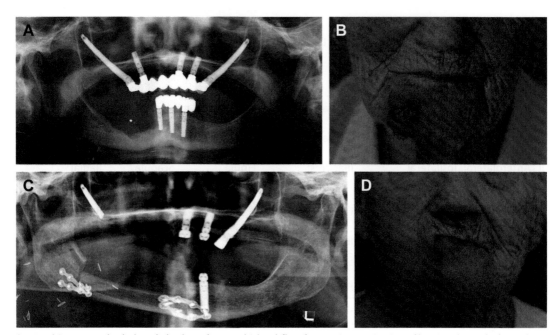

Fig. 3. This woman had already had a submental island flap for carcinoma-in-situ affecting the right buccal mucosa and then developed a far more aggressive squamous cell carcinoma invading the mandible and the mental skin. (*A*) Preoperative orthopantomogram shows a squamous cell carcinoma causing bone loss in the right premolar region. Note the previous rehabilitation with zygomatic and piriform implants to retain an upper full denture. (*B*) Facial view showing invasion of the facial skin. (*C*, *D*) In this case it was possible to reconstruct the mandible in a more posterior position allowing the closure of the facial skin and fibula skin used intraorally.

Irrespective of the flap option, be careful not to faithfully reconstruct the size of the mandible especially in edentulous or partially dentate patients. The maxilla tends to lose bone in an anteroposterior direction becoming more posterior in position compared with the facial tissues. In the mandible bone is lost from superior to inferior so that the jaw remains in the same facial

Table 2
Flap type preference related to the extent and type of maxillectomy

Class	Preference Assuming No Skull Base Involvement			
	Most Preferred	**Second Best**	**Third Best**	**Least Preferred**
I (low maxillectomy not involving the maxillary sinus)	Local flap unless involving central hard palate when only soft tissue is required.			
II (Low maxillectomy not involving orbit or nasal bones)	Fibula and iliac crest equal merit unless high perinasal bone loss		Scapula tip	Radial
III (High maxillectomy including orbital floor but retaining orbit)	Iliac crest	Fibula	Scapula tip	Radial
IV (High maxillectomy and orbital exenteration)	Iliac crest and scapula tip equal merit for facial support (iliac best for dental rehabilitation)		Fibula	Radial
V (Orbitomaxillary [not including alveolus])	Radial, perforator flap (long pedicle) equal merit. Bone transfer is not an advantage			
VI (Nasomaxillary [not including alveolus])	Radial	Scapula tip	Soft tissue flaps increase risk of nasal collapse	

Class I cases are unlikely to need reconstruction because a partial dental prosthesis can effectively deal with the alveolar defect.

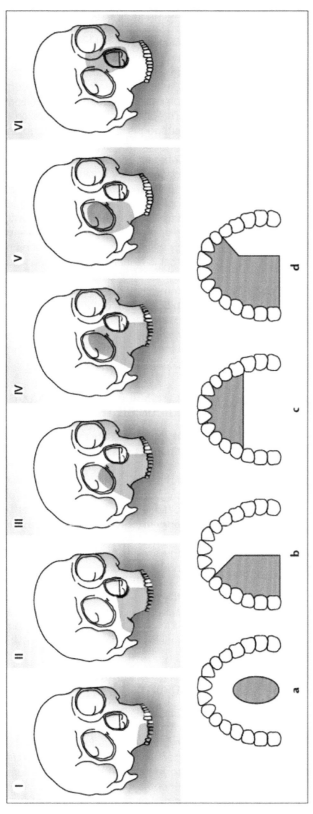

Fig. 4. Classification. Class I–IV (vertical component of maxillectomy). Class I: alveolus but not maxillary sinus; Class II: low maxillectomy not involving the orbit or nasal bone; Class III: high maxillectomy involving orbital floor but retaining orbit; Class IV: high maxillectomy including the orbit. The horizontal elements of the defect: a, not involving talveolus; b, less than half alveolus; c, anterior bilateral but less than half alveolus; d, bilateral greater than half alveolus. Class V: orbitomaxillary (no alveolar bone). Class VI: nasomaxillary (no alveolar bone). (*From* Brown JS, Barry C, Ho MW, et al. A new classification for mandibular defects after oncological resection. Lancet Oncol 2016;17(1):e23–30; with permission.)

position, which means it is generally advisable to reconstruct in a more posterior position for the mandible (**Fig. 3**). This has advantages because the oral tissues and the facial envelope are under less tension, and a likely improved facial profile.

AVOIDING POOR RESULTS AFTER SUCCESSFUL FLAP TRANSFER FOR RECONSTRUCTION OF THE MAXILLA AND MIDFACE

It is clear in the literature and from my own experience that reconstructing the maxilla and midface is complex and there are several suggestions of how best to achieve optimum results for the patient.[20–22] **Table 2** summarizes the Liverpool ethos toward maxillary and midface defect reconstruction based on the *Lancet* classification (**Fig. 4**).[23]

CLASS I (LOW-LEVEL MAXILLECTOMY NOT INVOLVING MAXILLARY SINUS)

Free tissue transfer is generally not needed for class I defects because these do not cause an oroantral fistula if laterally located. If the defect is central, however, then it may be advantageous to reconstruct the loss on the nondental part of the hard palate but only a soft tissue flap is needed (**Fig. 5**).

CLASS II (LOW-LEVEL MAXILLECTOMY NOT INVOLVING THE ORBITAL OR NASAL BONES)

Similarly there is good evidence that with implant-retained obturation excellent results are obtained for all class II defects not involving the orbit.[24] These should be considered carefully with the maxillofacial prosthodontist and due discussion with the wishes of the patient and family. These are relatively low defects with little change to the external appearance or the orbit and so the main

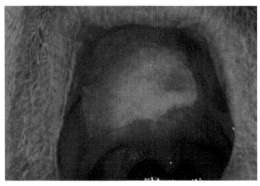

Fig. 5. Class I defect not involving the dental-bearing alveolus reconstructed with a radial forearm flap.

factor to be restored is the dentition to enable adequate chewing and dental appearance. The advantage of obturation from the start is that the final result is achieved more rapidly. Although immediate implants can be placed at the time a free flap is placed, the orientation and usefulness are limited unless significant computed tomography–based preoperative planning is undertaken.[25] The choice of flap depends on how much nasal support is lost in the resection and the placement of implants with a favorable implant/soft tissue interface is often improved with a muscle as opposed to a skin flap. Excellent results are achievable with fibula and iliac crest with internal oblique but there is definitely a place for soft tissue flap reconstruction together with the immediate placement of zygomatic implants (**Fig. 6**). In our practice the scapula tip[26] does not provide bone that is reliably implanted and would be an unlikely choice in a similar way to the composite radial forearm. If the patient had an unfavorable comorbidity, then obturation with immediate implant placement is our preferred option. A definitive bar retained obturator prosthesis is usually provided within 2 weeks in an immediately loaded prosthodontic protocol.

CLASS III (HIGH-LEVEL MAXILLECTOMY RETAINING THE ORBIT)

If there is no substantial loss of overlying skin then the most satisfactory reconstruction that can provide adequate bone for implants, good support for the orbital floor reconstruction, and a satisfactory long-term result is the iliac crest with internal oblique muscle.[27,28] I have not used the scapula tip with teres major, latissimus dorsi muscle, or serratus anterior for the class III defect mainly because the bone is not sufficient to take implants reliably and longer term results have been disappointing. Most of these patients require postoperative radiotherapy for squamous cell resection and the blood supply to the iliac crest through the deep circumflex iliac artery and the ascending branch ensure reliable healing and reduces the risk of nonunion.

CLASS IV (HIGH-LEVEL MAXILLECTOMY AND ORBIT)

This defect includes the removal of part of the dental alveolus and the maxilla, and includes an orbital exenteration. This means that there is no need to provide reliable support for the orbital floor to reduce the risk of contracture, ectropion, and enopthalmos, which greatly simplifies the reconstruction and opens the options. Much depends on whether prosthetic and prosthodontic

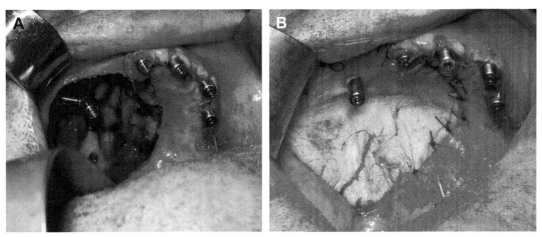

Fig. 6. A patient requiring a class IId defect reconstructed with the combination of a radial forearm flap to close the oronasal fistula and immediate implants including a zygomatic implant on the left side. (*A*) Defect and immediate implants placed. (*B*) Radial forearm flap used to close the oronasal fistula and provide an ideal interface between the implant and prosthesis.

rehabilitation is planned for the oral cavity and orbit and we still favor the iliac crest with internal oblique, which provides an excellent orbital cavity and enough good bone for an implant-retained upper denture. Without the need for a full or partial upper denture then other options can work well, although the fibula provides little appropriate soft tissue in the orbital region.

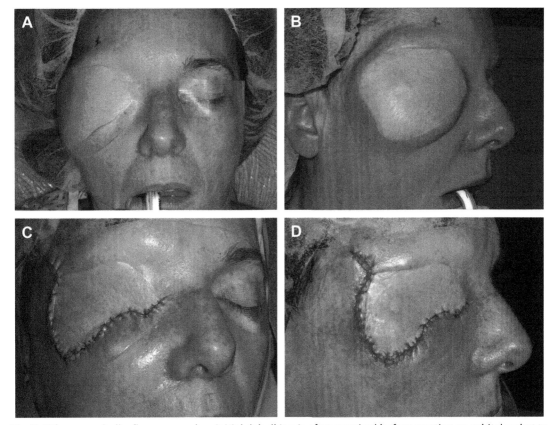

Fig. 7. Where very bulky flaps are used an initial debulking is often required before creating an orbital socket to accommodate the prosthesis. (*A, B*) Class V defect reconstruction with latissimus dorsi flap. (*C, D*) Postdebulking.

CLASS V (ORBITOMAXILLARY)

With the loss of the eye a prosthesis must be considered unless the patient is happy with a patch. If a prosthesis is planned then it is advantageous not to fill the orbit so as to allow space for the prosthesis to be placed, often with the benefit of implants. There is no need to restore the bone contour because this can be restored with the prosthesis if the patient prefers. Once again the whole reconstruction is simplified because the alveolus and dentition remain intact; there is little need for facial nerve function except the mandibular branch often unaffected with this resection. It is really up to the choice of the surgeon working closely with the maxillofacial prosthetist (**Fig. 7**).

CLASS VI (NASOMAXILLARY)

This defect includes the standard rhinectomy, which is easily replaced with prosthesis if appropriate anchorage is planned at the time of the resection. In our unit we favor the use of immediate horizontally placed zygomatic implants allowing for early loading of the prosthesis in function (**Fig. 8**). However, problems may arise when the resection is higher and includes the skin and bone separating the orbits. In this situation the lower part of the nose, sometimes including the alar region, can be retained, leaving a complex reconstruction. I take the composite radial forearm flap as my first option and I have included a case in the *Lancet* article in 2010,[23] which shows this principle very well. We have tried the scapula tip and latissimus dorsi muscle and overlying skin graft but this did not work well. It is essential to include a specialist oculoplastic surgeon in the resection and reconstruction to give the best chance of retaining a functioning lacrimal system on both sides. These cases emphasize the importance of a multidisciplinary approach for all head and neck reconstructive surgery.

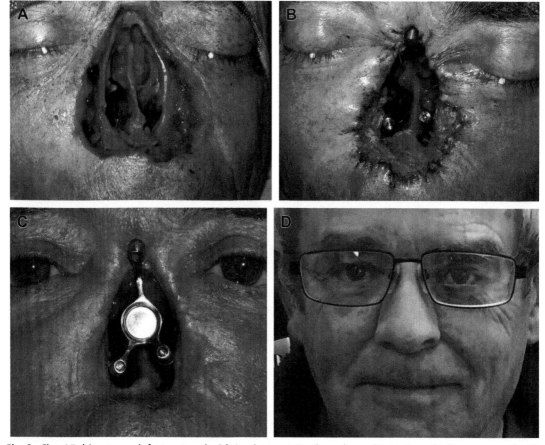

Fig. 8. Class VI rhinectomy defect restored with implant, retained nasal prosthesis. Note the importance of split-skin grafting to nasal floor and lateral aspects of the defect. (*A*) Postrhinectomy defect. (*B*) Immediate implants have been placed. (*C*) Implant-retained structure designed to hold the prosthesis. (*D*) Final result showing full nasal prosthesis.

SUMMARY

Microvascular reconstructive surgery requires a combined approach with sufficient number of cases and complexity to develop into a team to cover midface and maxilla and oral/oropharyngeal soft tissue and mandibular reconstruction. Short-term results are often reliable but be prepared to look at longer term results (greater than 2 years) when, after radiotherapy, less substantial and well-vascularized reconstructions may start to fail.

REFERENCES

1. Shaw RJ, Kanatas AN, Lowe D, et al. Comparison of miniplates and reconstruction plates in mandibular reconstruction. Head Neck 2004;26:456–63.

2. Brown JS, Magennis P, Rogers SN, et al. Trends in head and neck microvascular reconstructive surgery in Liverpool (1992-2001). Br J Oral Maxillofac Surg 2006;44:364–70.

3. Brown JS, Rogers SN, Lowe D. A comparison of tongue and soft palate squamous cell carcinoma treated by primary surgery in terms of survival and quality of life outcomes. Int J Oral Maxillofac Surg 2006;35:208–14.

4. Brown JS, Thomas S, Chakrabati A, et al. Patient preference in placement for the donor site scar in head and neck reconstruction. Plast Reconstr Surg 2008;122:20e–2e.

5. Brown JS, Barry C, Ho MW, et al. A new classification for mandibular defects after oncological resection. Lancet Oncol 2016;17(1):e23–30.

6. Shaw RJ, Brown JS. Osteomyocutaneous deep circumflex artery perforator flap in the reconstruction of midface defect with facial skin loss: a case report. Microsurgery 2009;29(4):299–302.

7. Shaw RJ, Ho MW, Brown JS. Thoracodorsal artery perforator flap in oromandibular reconstruction with associated large facial skin defects. Br J Oral Maxillofac Surg 2015;53(6):569–71.

8. Fernandes R. Local and regional flaps in head and neck reconstruction. Danvers (MA): Wiley Blackwell; 2015. p. 147–61, 162–9.

9. Hara I, Gellrich NC, Duke J, et al. Swallowing and speech function after intraoral soft tissue reconstruction with lateral upper arm free flap and radial forearm free flap. Br J Oral Maxillofac Surg 2003;41(3):161–9.

10. Wei FC, Jain V, Celik N, et al. Have we found an ideal soft-tissue flap? An experience with 672 anterolateral thigh flaps. Plast Reconstr Surg 2002;109(7):2219–26.

11. Wolff KD, Bauer F, Kunz S, et al. Superficial lateral sural artery perforator flap for intraoral reconstruction: anatomical study and clinical implications. Head Neck 2012;34(9):1218–24.

12. Nugent M, Endersby S, Kennedy M, et al. Early experience with the medial sural artery perforator flap as an alternative to the radial forearm flap for reconstruction in the head and neck. Br J Oral Maxillofac Surg 2015;53(5):461–3.

13. Steiner W, Fierek O, Ambrosch P, et al. Transoral laser microsurgery for squamous cell carcinoma of the posterior tongue. Arch Otolaryngol Head Neck Surg 2003;129(1):36–43.

14. Brown JS, Zuydam AC, Jones DC, et al. Functional outcome in soft palate reconstruction using a radial forearm free flap in conjunction with a superiorly based pharyngeal flap. Head Neck 1997;19:524–34.

15. Cordeiro PG, Disa JJ, Hidalgo D, et al. Reconstruction of the mandible with osseous free flaps: a 10-year experience with 150 consecutive patients. Plast Reconstr Surg 1999;104(5):1314–20.

16. Rogers SN, Lkasmiah S, Narayan B, et al. A comparison of long-term morbidity following deep circumflex iliac and fibula free flaps for reconstruction following head and neck cancer. Plast Reconstr Surg 2003;112(6):1517–25.

17. Richardson D, Fisher SE, Vaughan ED, et al. Radial forearm flap donor-site complications and morbidity: a prospective study. Plast Reconstr Surg 1997;99:109–15.

18. Villaret DB, Futran NA. The indications and outcomes of the use of osteocutaneous radial forearm flap. Head Neck 2003;25(6):475–81.

19. Cawood JI, Howell RA. A classification of the edentulous jaws. Int J Oral Maxillofac Surg 1988;17(4):2332–6.

20. Santamaria E, Cordeiro PG. Reconstruction of maxillectomy and midfacial defect with free tissue transfer. J Surg Oncol 2006;94:522–31.

21. Brown JS, Rogers SN, McNally DN, et al. A modified classification for the maxillectomy defect. Head Neck 2000;22(1):17–26.

22. Hanasano MM, Silva AK, Yu P, et al. A comprehensive algorithm for oncologic maxillary reconstruction. Plast Reconstr Surg 2013;13(1):47–60.

23. Brown JS, Shaw RJ. Reconstruction of the maxilla and midface: introducing a new classification. Lancet Oncol 2010;11(10):1001–8.

24. Boyes-Varley JG, Howes DG, Davidge-Pitts KD, et al. A protocol for maxillary reconstruction following oncology resection using zygomatic implants. Int J Prosthodont 2007;20(5):521–31.

25. Fenlon MR, Lyons A, Farrell S, et al. Factors affecting survival and usefulness of implants laced in vascularised free composite grafts in post-head and neck cancer reconstruction. Clin Implant Dent Relat Res 2012;14(2):266–72.

26. Clark JR, Vesely M, Gilbert R. Scapula angle osteo-myogenous flap in postmaxillectomy reconstruction: defect, reconstruction, shoulder function, and harvest technique. Head Neck 2008;30(1):10–20.

27. Brown JS. Deep circumflex iliac artery free flap with internal oblique muscle as a new method of immediate reconstruction of maxillectomy defect. Head Neck 1996;18:412–21.

28. Brown JS. Reconstruction of the maxilla with loss of the orbital floor and orbital preservation: a case for the iliac crest with internal oblique. Semin Plast Surg 2008;22(3):161–74.

Lessons Learned from Delayed Versus Immediate Microsurgical Reconstruction of Complex Maxillectomy and Midfacial Defects

Experience in a Tertiary Center in Mexico

Eric Santamaria, MD[a],*, Erika de la Concha, MD[b]

KEYWORDS

- Maxillectomy • Free flaps • Radiotherapy • Head and neck reconstruction
- Immediate reconstruction • Delayed reconstruction

KEY POINTS

- Free flaps have become the first option for reconstruction of maxillectomy and midfacial defects, with successful functional and aesthetic outcomes, particularly when performed immediately.
- Delayed reconstruction of maxillectomy defects is associated with significantly higher rates of complication probably secondary to radiotherapy and recurrent infections from long-term oral or nasal cavity communication.
- Therefore, multiple free and local flaps are required in this group of patients to address wound dehiscence with hardware exposure, orocutaneous fistula, and upper lip or partial nasal retraction and to provide stable skeletal and soft tissue reconstruction.

INTRODUCTION

Reconstruction of maxillectomy and midfacial defects are among the most challenging procedures in plastic surgery. Defects in this anatomic area frequently have suboptimal aesthetic and functional outcomes, affecting speech, oral competence, eye globe position and function, among others.[1–3] Microsurgical free tissue transfer is currently the treatment of choice for the reconstruction of complex midfacial defects.[1] The overall success rate of microsurgical transfer of tissue in the head and neck is reported to be more than 90%.[4] Various factors and patients' characteristics have been identified as having an influence in the outcome of microsurgical reconstruction.[5,6]

This article has not been presented previously at any meeting or conference.
Disclosures: The authors have nothing to disclose.
Patient Consent: Patients provided written consent for the use of their images.
[a] Department of Plastic and Reconstructive Surgery, Hospital General Dr. Manuel Gea Gonzalez, National Cancer Institute, Universidad Nacional Autonoma de Mexico, Av. Calzada de Tlalpan 4800, Tlalpan, Sección XVI, 14080 Ciudad de México, Mexico; [b] Department of Plastic and Reconstructive Surgery, Hospital General Dr. Manuel Gea Gonzalez, Av. Calzada de Tlalpan 4800, Tlalpan, Sección XVI, 14080 Ciudad de México, Mexico
* Corresponding author.
E-mail address: ericsanta@prodigy.net.mx

Clin Plastic Surg 43 (2016) 719–727
http://dx.doi.org/10.1016/j.cps.2016.05.011

Apart from patients' medical conditions, preoperative treatment with radiotherapy is one of the main factors that influences postoperative outcomes.[7,8] The introduction of radiotherapy has resulted in increased survival of patients diagnosed with head and neck malignancies; therefore, current treatment involves a combination of surgical resection with either immediate or delayed reconstruction and radiotherapy.[9,10]

In the year 2000, Cordeiro and Santamaria[2] published a classification system and algorithm for reconstruction of maxillectomy and midfacial defects. Flap selection was determined by the type of bony resection and missing soft tissue volume and skin surface and is described as follows: type I, limited maxillectomy; type II, subtotal maxillectomy; type IIIa, total maxillectomy with preservation of orbital contents; type IIIb, total maxillectomy with orbital exenteration; and type IV, orbitomaxillectomy. This classification system helps to determine the best approach for microsurgical free flap reconstruction based on the type of defect.

The objective of this article is to describe the common pitfalls encountered in delayed and immediate microsurgical reconstruction of complex maxillectomy and midfacial defects. The authors present the most commonly used free flaps, complications, and functional and aesthetic outcomes in complex midfacial reconstruction in a tertiary center in Mexico.

METHODS

Over a 16-year period (1999–2015), 37 patients were reconstructed for complex midfacial defects using 52 free flaps that were performed by a single surgeon (E.S.) at a tertiary center, Hospital General Dr Manuel Gea Gonzalez, in Mexico City. The authors conducted a retrospective chart review to record demographic data, reconstructive procedures, and complications and compared the functional and aesthetic outcomes between delayed and immediate reconstruction groups. The measurements were exported to the Statistical Package for Social Sciences (IBM SPSS Statistics 23.0) for statistical analyses. The differences in the immediate and delayed reconstruction groups were compared using a 2-sample t test, with a 95% confidence level. P values less than .05 were considered significant. The institutional review board of Hospital General Dr Manuel Gea Gonzalez approved this study.

RESULTS

A total of 37 patients were included in this study (immediate reconstruction group: 13, delayed reconstruction group: 24). The diagnoses of each group are presented in **Table 1**. The average patient age was 52 years (range 35–68 years) and 44 years (range 23–71 years) in the immediate and delayed reconstruction group, respectively. Patient characteristics and demographics are presented in **Table 2**. No statistically significant differences were observed between both groups regarding sex, smoking, diabetes, hypertension, and other comorbidities. The delayed reconstruction group had statistically significant ($P = .003$) more preoperative radiotherapy (66.7%) than the immediate reconstruction group (15%).

Types of free flaps used for reconstruction of midfacial defects based on the authors' classification system described in 2000[9] are listed in **Table 3**. The most commonly used was the fibula osteocutaneous free flap (n = 24), followed by the rectus abdominis myocutaneous free flap (n = 15). In contrast to the authors' previous algorithm treatment, the radial forearm osteocutaneous and fasciocutaneous free flaps were rarely used (n = 6). In addition to using multiple free flaps, some patients required one or more local flaps for reconstruction of complex structures, such as eyelids, lips, and nose. The delayed group required more local flaps for reconstruction of these complex structures (n = 12) compared with the immediate group (n = 4). These flaps included 9 forehead flaps for eyelids (n = 3) and partial nasal (n = 6) reconstruction, 3 lower lip to upper lip switch-flap procedures, 2 naso-labial flaps for partial nasal reconstruction, and 2 facial artery myomucosal flaps for upper lip inner lining.

A total of 52 free flaps were performed in 37 patients (**Table 4**). In the immediate reconstruction group (n = 13) only 3 patients required 2 free flaps to complete their reconstruction. Whereas, in the delayed group 8 patients required 2 free flaps and 2 patients required 3 free flaps. The most common combination of free flaps was fibula osteocutaneous free flap and a soft tissue free flap, to provide volume replacement and skin

Table 1		
Diagnosis of patients		
Diagnosis	Immediate Reconstruction n = 13 (%)	Delayed Reconstruction n = 24 (%)
Malignant tumor	8 (61.5)	16 (66.7)
Benign tumor	4 (30.8)	6 (25.0)
Trauma	1 (7.7)	2 (3.0)

Table 2
Patient characteristics

Patient Characteristics	Immediate Recon-struction (n = 13)	Delayed Recon-struction (n = 24)
Age (mean)	52 (range 35–68 y)	44 (range 23–71 y)
Sex:		
Male/female	9/4	16/8
Smoker	3	5
Diabetes	1	2
Hypertension	5	3
Radiotherapy[a]	2	16
Other comorbidities	2	2

[a] Statistically significant P = .003.

resurfacing either intraorally or for external coverage (ie, rectus abdominis or anterolateral thigh [ALT]).

Table 5 displays flap-related complications. In the immediate reconstruction group, 16 flaps were performed in 13 patients. In the delayed reconstruction group, 36 flaps were performed in 24 patients. Analysis of flap-related complications revealed a statistically significant higher wound dehiscence rate (P = .001) in the delayed reconstruction group (53%) compared with the immediate reconstruction group (6%). No differences in free flap re-exploration, partial and total flap loss, infection, and hematoma rates were observed. Average follow-up time was 53 months (range from 8 to 178) and 76 months (range from 10 to 126 months) for immediate and delayed reconstruction groups, respectively.

Functional and Aesthetic Outcomes

Functional and aesthetic outcomes are summarized in **Table 6**. In 34 patients who underwent resection of the palate, speech was rated normal in 23 patients (67%), nearly normal in 6 (18%), intelligible in 4 (12%), and finally unintelligible in 1 (3%). In the same group of patients with palatal resection, 27 patients (79%) were able to eat an unrestricted diet, 6 (18%) could manage a soft diet, 1 (3%) was able to tolerate liquids, and no patients required a feeding tube. In this group, 30 patients (88%) had oral competence and 7 patients (21%) presented a palatal fistula postoperatively. Eighty-five percent of patients with postoperative fistula (n = 6) belonged to the delayed reconstruction group (see **Table 6**).

Table 3
Types of flaps used for reconstruction

Maxillectomy Defect Type	No. of Patients	No. of Free Flaps	Rectus Abdominis Myocutaneous	Radial Forearm Fascio-Cutaneous	Radial Forearm Osteo-Cutaneous	Fibula Osteo-Cutaneous	ALT	Other (Local Flaps)[a]
Immediate reconstruction								
I	2	2	—	2	—	—	—	—
II	3	3	—	—	1	2	—	—
IIIa	7	10	2	—	—	5	3	3
IIIb	1	1	1	—	—	—	—	1
IV	0	0	—	—	—	—	—	—
Total	13	16	3	2	1	7	3	4
Delayed reconstruction								—
I	1	1	—	1	—	—	—	—
II	4	4	—	—	1	3	—	1
IIIa	16	27	9	1	—	13	4	10
IIIb	1	1	1	—	—	—	—	1
IV	2	3	2	—	—	1	—	—
Total	24	36	12	2	1	17	4	12
Total	*37*	*52*	*15*	*4*	*2*	*24*	*7*	*16*

Abbreviation: ALT, anterolateral thigh.
[a] Local flaps included 9 forehead flaps for eyelids (3) and partial nasal (6) reconstruction, 3 lower lip to upper lip switch-flap procedures, 2 nasolabial flap for partial nasal reconstruction, and 2 facial artery myo-mucosal flaps for upper lip inner lining.

Table 4
Number of flaps performed per patient

Reconstructive Surgeries	Total Free Flaps	1 Free Flap per Patient	2 Free Flaps per Patient	3 Free Flaps per Patient	Total Secondary Local Flaps	1 Secondary Local Flap	2 Secondary Local Flaps
Immediate reconstruction (n = 13)	16	10	3	0	4	2	1
Delayed reconstruction (n = 24)	36	14	8	2	12	4	4
Total	52	24	11	2	16	6	5

Twenty-four patients underwent resection of the orbital floor (23 patients with defects type IIIa and 1 patient with type I maxillectomy) and were assessed for eye globe position and function. Normal vision was found in 17 patients (71%). Patients developed either one or multiple complications due to eye globe malposition: ectropion was observed in 8 patients (33%), enophthalmos in 3 patients (12%), dystopia in 3 patients (12%), and diplopia in 4 patients (17%) (see **Table 6**).

Aesthetic outcomes were assessed in all 37 patients 6 months after completing maxillectomy reconstruction. Eleven patients were evaluated as having excellent results (84%) in the immediate reconstruction group (**Fig. 1**) and only 5 in the delayed group (21%). One patient had good results in the immediate group (8%) compared with 9 patients in the delayed group (38%); one patient had fair results in the immediate group (8%) versus 6 in the delayed group (25%); finally, 4 patients had poor results in the delayed group (16%) with none in the immediate group (**Fig. 2**).

DISCUSSION

Reconstruction of maxillary and midfacial defects after resection of tumors or trauma has changed dramatically in recent years. The use of an intraoral prosthetic obturator is indicated only in patients who are not candidates for reconstruction with autologous tissue and, in particular, with free flaps, which is considered the gold standard technique for functional reconstruction of the maxilla.

The main objectives of maxillectomy and midfacial reconstruction are to enable patients to proper speech, chewing, and swallowing. In addition, when the orbital content is spared, it is mandatory to avoid diplopia. For more radical defects, sometimes it is required to obliterate communications between the maxillary sinus and the nasal cavity or the skull base. From the cosmetic point of view, the aim is to restore the skeletal support provided by the maxilla and, when required, to replace the overlying soft tissues, including important functional structures, such as the eyelids and oral sphincter. Immediate reconstruction is always preferable, in order to minimize complications, such as fistulas, oronasal regurgitation, eye globe displacement, scarring contraction, infections and wound-healing problems, especially when the tumor resection is followed by postoperative radiotherapy. Unfortunately, not every patient has the opportunity to receive immediate reconstruction. In the authors' center, for instance, most patients are referred to them from the National Cancer Institute, after they underwent maxillectomy and

Table 5
Complications

Timing of Reconstruction	No. of Cases	No. of Free Flaps	No. of Free Flap Re-exploration n (%)	Partial Flap Loss n (%)	Free Flap Loss n (%)	Wound Dehiscence n (%)[a]	Infection n (%)	Hematoma n (%)
Immediate	13	16	1 (6.0)	0 (0)	0 (0)	1 (6)	0 (0)	0 (0)
Delayed	24	36	3 (8.0)	2 (5.0)	1 (3.0)	19 (53)	6 (16)	1 (3.0)
Total	37	52	4 (7.6)	2 (3.8)	1 (1.9)	20 (38)	6 (11)	1 (1.9)

[a] Statistically significant P = .001.

Table 6
Functional and aesthetic outcomes

	Immediate Reconstruction n = 13 (%)	Delayed Reconstruction n = 21 (%)	Total n = 34 (%)
Speech[a]			
Normal	10 (77)	13 (62)	23 (67)
Nearly normal	2 (15)	4 (19)	6 (18)
Intelligible	1 (8)	3 (14)	4 (12)
Unintelligible	0	1 (5)	1 (3)
Diet[a]			
Unrestricted	11 (85)	16 (76)	27 (79)
Soft	2 (15)	4 (19)	6 (18)
Liquids	0	1 (5)	1 (3)
Feeding tube	0	0	0
Oral competence[a]			
Yes	13 (100)	17 (81)	30 (88)
No	0	4 (19)	4 (12)
Palatal fistula[a]			
Yes	1 (8)	6 (29)	7 (21)
No	12 (92)	15 (71)	27 (79)
	Immediate Reconstruction n = 7 (%)	Delayed Reconstruction n = 17 (%)	Total n = 24 (%)
Eye globe position and function[b]			
Normal	5 (71)	12 (70)	17 (71)
Ectropion	3 (43)	5 (29)	8 (33)
Enophthalmos	0	3 (18)	3 (12)
Dystopia	1 (14)	2 (12)	3 (12)
Diplopia	1 (14)	3 (18)	4 (17)
	Immediate Reconstruction n = 13 (%)	Delayed Reconstruction n = 24 (%)	Total n = 37 (%)
Aesthetic results[c]			
Excellent	11 (84)	5 (21)	16 (43)
Good	1 (8)	9 (38)	10 (27)
Fair	1 (8)	6 (25)	7 (19)
Poor	0	4 (16)	4 (11)

[a] Assessed only in type II, IIIa, IIIb, and 2 patients with partial (type I) maxillectomy defect.
[b] Assessed only in all type IIIa and 1 patient with partial (type I) maxillectomy defect. Multiple complications coexisted in some patients.
[c] Assessed in all types of maxillectomy defects.

adjuvant therapy when indicated. From this experience, the authors learned how challenging delayed reconstruction of maxillectomy and midfacial defects can be and how to address the multiple complications they observed in this group of patients when compared with immediate reconstruction.

Unlike the authors' classification system and reconstructive algorithm described in 2000[2] in which all of their patients had postoncological

resection defects and were reconstructed immediately, in this article, they include patients with benign conditions and delayed reconstructions. The authors also include patients that were reconstructed using other flaps, such as the fibula osteocutaneous and the ALT free flap. For external skin and soft tissue volume reconstruction, the radial forearm flap used to be the first choice. However, this flap is usually too thin for adequate coverage of bone grafts and plates, provides

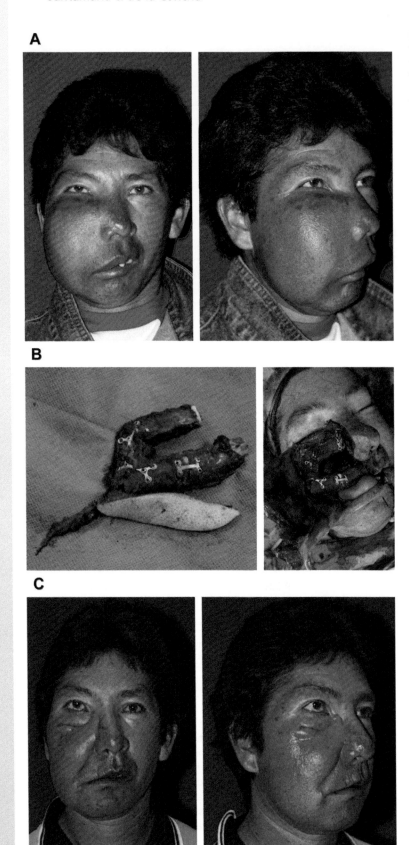

Fig. 1. Immediate reconstruction of a total maxillectomy defect with preservation of the orbital contents (type IIIa) using a fibula osteocutaneous free flap. (*A*) Preoperative pictures of the patient. (*B*) Osteocutaneous fibula free flap with multiple osteotomies performed to recreate the horizontal and vertical buttresses of the maxilla. The distal part of the skin island was used for palatal resurfacing, and the proximal portion of the skin island was de-epithelialized for volume replacement and obliteration of the maxillary sinus. (*C*) Postoperative pictures of the patient.

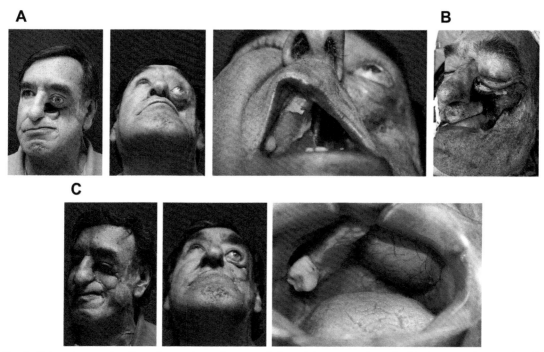

Fig. 2. Delayed reconstruction of a total maxillectomy defect with preservation of orbital content (type IIIa) with history of radiotherapy that was previously reconstructed using a skin graft and obturator prosthesis. (*A*) Preoperative pictures of the patient. (*B*) Orbital content support was provided with split rib graft; a 3 skin-islands vertical rectus abdominis myocutaneous free flap was used to reconstruct nasal cavity, palatal surface, and cheek coverage. (*C*) The patient developed postoperative infection and wound dehiscence due to nasal cavity fistula. The aesthetic and functional outcomes in this patient are poor and will require another free flap reconstruction.

insufficient volume replacement in extensive defects, sacrifices a major artery, and the morbidity in the donor site has led to a decrease in the use of this flap.[11] In recent years, the ALT free flap has replaced the use of the radial forearm flap because it is a reliable flap with less donor site morbidity.[12]

In contrast to the authors' previous report, in this study most patients were reconstructed with a fibula osteocutaneous free flap (n = 24). The rectus abdominis is still a good option; however, it does not provide any bone for skeletal framework. Several investigators have included the fibula osteocutaneous free flap into the armamentarium for reconstruction of maxillectomy and midfacial defects because it can replace bone and soft tissue defects in one stage.[10,13,14] In the authors' experience, the amount of soft tissue provided by this free flap is insufficient to provide enough volume to obliterate extensive dead spaces and soft tissue defects. In addition, it is difficult to design multiple skin islands to separate midfacial cavities and to provide simultaneously cheek external coverage when required. It is well recognized that soft tissue volume deficiencies are poorly tolerated in head and neck reconstruction.

Dead spaces should be obliterated to prevent accumulation of fluid that may cause secondary infection or presence of fistulas that lead to wound dehiscence and even compromise flap survival. Appropriate reconstruction is also important in prevention of bone and plate exposure.[15] Furthermore, whenever the skin island of a fibula osteocutaneous free flap is being used to replace gingival mucosa, the skin is very thick and requires multiple debulking procedures or replacement with palatal mucosal grafts before definitive placement of osseointegrated dental implants. For this reason, the authors previously described the prelaminated osteomucosal fibula flap for reconstruction of very small central maxillectomy defects (type I and II).[16] However, the authors did not include this group of patients in the present study because they underwent orthognathic osteotomies that could bias their comparative results.

From the authors' results analysis, it is evident that patients with delayed reconstruction had a greater number of complications than patients with immediate reconstruction and, therefore, required more free flaps and local flaps to obtain an acceptable functional and aesthetic outcome. This finding is similar to Gerressen and colleagues'[17] report, who described in 2013 that timing of reconstruction significantly affects flap survival, with primary reconstruction having higher success rates of free flaps than secondary reconstructions (94.8% vs 86.1% success rate with a $P = .0042$). Furthermore, the delayed reconstruction group presented more complications than the immediate group. Halle and colleagues[18] found similar results; they concluded that the largest increase in postoperative complications (ie, flap loss, delayed wound healing, wound infections) occurred if more than 6 weeks had passed since radiotherapy. These investigators advocate performing microsurgical reconstruction within 6 weeks of radiotherapy and suggest postoperative radiotherapy when possible. Preoperative radiotherapy is a widely acknowledged factor of local complications in different types of surgical procedures for the head and neck.[5,7,19] Ishimaru and colleagues[20] recently reported preoperative radiotherapy as a risk factor associated with free flap failure in a study of 2846 patients. Bourget and colleagues[21] reported an overall complication prevalence of 47% in 137 patients who had free tissue transferred to head and neck–irradiated fields, which is comparable with the authors' results. Benatar and colleagues[22] measured the impact on free flap success on local complications finding that preoperative radiotherapy was a significant risk factor for fistula formation and wound infection. Comparable with the authors' results, Preidl and colleagues[5] reported in 2015 that patients previously treated by irradiation required significantly more revision surgeries than those without radiotherapy.

The most common maxillectomy defects present in the authors' study were patients with total maxillectomy and preservation of the orbital contents (type IIIa). These patients also represented the most challenging group to reconstruct because they have more functional requirements: adequate ocular globe position, obliteration of any communication between the maxillary sinus and the palate or nasal cavity, and teeth restitution.[23] This group had the highest number of palatal fistulas, wound dehiscence, and vision problems and the worst results in speech, mastication, and ocular function. This finding correlates to several investigators' reports, like Benatar and colleagues[22] who found that reconstruction with an osteocutaneous flap in patients with oral defects was also a significant risk factor for local complications.

Hanasono and colleagues[24] reported in 2014 that multiple sequential free flaps in a patient for reconstruction in head and neck are feasible and reliable; they should be intended to improve patient aesthetics and function or in cases of recurrent cancers. Sequential free flaps should be attempted rather than a less-than-desirable reconstruction in a one-stage procedure.

In the authors' experience, they recommend immediate reconstruction of maxillectomy defects whenever possible. Nevertheless, in patients who are candidates for delayed reconstruction with a history of radiotherapy, they suggest using first a nonvascularized bone graft for the orbital floor and a soft tissue free flap to obliterate the defect and seal communications with the oral cavity, nasal cavity, and, in some cases, with the skull base. Afterward, in a second stage, reconstruct the bony framework with an osseous free flap for placement of osseointegrated dental implants. The fibula free flap should be reserved as a first option in cases of immediate reconstruction for type II and IIIa defects. In cases of delayed reconstruction, this free flap should be reserved for patients with defects due to a benign condition or trauma with no side effects from radiotherapy.

SUMMARY

Free flaps have become the first option for reconstruction of maxillectomy and midfacial defects, with successful functional and aesthetic outcomes, particularly when performed immediately.

Delayed reconstruction of maxillectomy defects is associated with significantly higher rates of complication probably secondary to radiotherapy and recurrent infections from long-term oral or nasal cavity communication. Therefore, multiple free and local flaps are required in this group of patients to address wound dehiscence with hardware exposure, orocutaneous fistula, and upper lip or partial nasal retraction and to provide stable skeletal and soft tissue reconstruction.

REFERENCES

1. Cordeiro PG, Chen CM. A 15-year review of midface reconstruction after total and subtotal maxillectomy: part I. Algorithm and outcomes. Plast Reconstr Surg 2012;129(1):124–36.
2. Cordeiro PG, Santamaria E. A classification system and algorithm for reconstruction of maxillectomy and midfacial defects. Plast Reconstr Surg 2000; 105(7):2331–46.
3. Cordeiro PG, Chen CM. A 15-year review of midface reconstruction after total and subtotal maxillectomy: Part II. Technical modifications to maximize aesthetic and functional outcomes. Plast Reconstr Surg 2012;129(1):139–47.
4. Pohlenz P, Blessmann M, Blake F, et al. Outcome and complications of 540 microvascular free flaps: the Hamburg experience. Clin Oral Investig 2007; 11:89–92.

5. Preidl RH, Wehrhan F, Schlittenbauser T, et al. Perioperative factor that influence the outcome of microsurgical reconstructions in craniomaxillofacial surgery. Br J Oral Maxillofac Surg 2015;53(6):533–7.

6. Singh B, Cordeiro PG, Santamaria E, et al. Factors associated with complications in microvascular reconstruction of head and neck defects. Plast Reconstr Surg 1999;103(2):403–11.

7. Mucke T, Rau A, Weitz J, et al. Influence of irradiation and oncologic surgery on head and neck microsurgical reconstructions. Oral Oncol 2012;48(4):367–71.

8. Momeni A, Kim FY, Kattan A, et al. The effect of preoperative radiotherapy on complication rate after microsurgical head and neck reconstruction. J Plast Reconstr Aesthet Surg 2011;64(11):1454–9.

9. Klug C, Berzaczy D, Reinbacher H, et al. Influence of previous radiotherapy on free tissue transfer in the head and neck region: evaluation of 455 cases. Laryngoscope 2006;116:1162–7.

10. Wennerberg J. Pre versus post-operative radiotherapy of resectable squamous cell carcinoma of the head and neck. Acta Otolaryngol 1995;115:465–74.

11. Wei FC, Yazar S, Lin CH, et al. Double free flaps in head and neck reconstruction. Clin Plast Surg 2005;32(3):303–8.

12. Wei FC, Celik N, Chen HC, et al. Combined anterolateral thigh flap and vascularized fibula osteoseptocutaneous flap in reconstruction of extensive composite mandibular defects. Plast Reconstr Surg 2002;109:45–52.

13. Sun J, Shen Y, Li J, et al. Reconstruction of high maxillectomy defects with the fibula osteomyocutaneous flap in combination with titanium mesh or a zygomatic implant. Plast Reconstr Surg 2011;127(1):150–60.

14. Futran ND, Wadsworth JT, Villaret D, et al. Midface reconstruction with fibula free flap. Arch Otolaryngol Head Neck Surg 2002;128:161–6.

15. Chen HC, Demirkan F, Wei FC, et al. Free fibula osteoseptocutaneous-pedicles pectoralis major myocutaneous flap combination in reconstruction of extensive composite mandibular defects. Plast Reconstr Surg 1999;103:839–45.

16. Santamaria E, Correa S, Bluebond-Langner R, et al. A shift from the osteocutaenous fibula flap to the prelaminated osteomucosal fibula flap for maxillary reconstruction. Plast Reconstr Surg 2012;130(5):1023–30.

17. Gerressen M, Pastashek CI, Riediger D, et al. Microsurgical free flap reconstructions of head and neck region in 406 cases: a 13 year experience. J Oral Maxillofac Surg 2013;71(3):628–35.

18. Halle M, Bodin I, Tornvall P, et al. Timing of radiotherapy in head and neck free flap reconstruction- a study of postoperative complications. J Plast Reconstr Aesthet Surg 2009;62:889–95.

19. Hanasono MM, Barnea Y, Skoracki RJ. Microvascular surgery in the previously operated and irradiated neck. Microsurgery 2009;29:1–7.

20. Ishimaru M, Ono S, Suzuki S, et al. Risk factors for free flap failure in 2,846 patients with head and neck cancer: a national database study in Japan. J Oral Maxillofac Surg 2016;74(6):1265–70.

21. Bourget A, Chang JT, Wu DB, et al. Free flap reconstruction in the head and neck region following radiotherapy; a cohort study identifying negative outcome predictors. Plast Reconstr Surg 2011;127:1901–8.

22. Benatar MJ, Dassonvile O, Chamorey E, et al. Impact of preoperative radiotherapy on head and neck free flap reconstruction: a report on 429 cases. J Plast Reconstr Aesthet Surg 2013;66(4):478–82.

23. Cordeiro PG, Santamaria E, Kraus DH, et al. Reconstruction of total maxillectomy defects with preservation of orbital contents. Plast Reconstr Surg 1998;102(6):1874–84.

24. Hanasono MM, Corbitt CA, Yu P, et al. Success of sequential free flaps in head and neck reconstruction. J Plast Reconstr Aesthet Surg 2014;67(9):1186–93.

Lessons Learned from Unfavorable Microsurgical Head and Neck Reconstruction
Japan National Cancer Center Hospital and Okayama University Hospital

Yoshihiro Kimata, MD[a],*, Hiroshi Matsumoto, MD[a],
Narusi Sugiyama, MD[a], Satoshi Onoda, MD[a],
Minoru Sakuraba, MD[b]

KEYWORDS

- Postoperative complications • Surgical site infection • Microvascular head and neck reconstruction
- Strategies for complications • Unfavorable result cases

KEY POINTS

- The risk of surgical site infection (SSI) remains high after major reconstructive surgery of the head and neck. The authors describe their clinical data regarding SSI in microsurgical tongue reconstruction at National Cancer Hospital in Japan.
- The relationship between SSI and preoperative irradiation at Okayama University Hospital in Japan was described. The data indicated a poor response to local infection in patients receiving chemotherapy or radiotherapy.
- Strategies for SSI control in head and neck reconstruction were described.

Various defects in the head and neck region have been successfully reconstructed with the development of microsurgical techniques. However the risk of local postoperative complications, including surgical site infection (SSI), still remains high after major reconstructive surgeries in the head and neck area. This high rate of complications is probably because of the complex anatomy of this area, the effect of preoperative cancer treatment, and the contamination of the intraoral and pharynx environment. In this article, the authors describe their clinical data concerning SSI in microsurgical tongue reconstruction at the National Cancer Hospital in Japan, unfavorable representative cases, the relationship between SSI and preoperative irradiation at Okayama University Hospital in Japan, and the strategy of control for SSI in head and neck reconstruction.

SURGICAL SITE INFECTION IN HEAD AND NECK RECONSTRUCTION

Head and neck cancer surgery is categorized as a clean-contaminated surgery by the Centers for

Disclosure Statement: There are no conflicts of interest to declare.
[a] Department of Plastic and Reconstructive Surgery, Okayama University, Graduate School of Medicine, Dentistry and Pharmaceutical Sciences, Okayama University, 2-5-1 Shikata-cho, Kita-ku, Okayama City, Okayama 700-8558, Japan; [b] Division of Head and Neck Surgery, National Cancer Center Hospital East, 6-5-1 Kashiwanoha, Kashiwa, Chiba 277-8577, Japan
* Corresponding author.
E-mail address: ykimata@cc.okayama-u.ac.jp

Clin Plastic Surg 43 (2016) 729–737
http://dx.doi.org/10.1016/j.cps.2016.05.002

Disease Control and Prevention.[1] However, the rate of SSI in head and neck surgeries is high compared with that in other clean-contaminated surgeries. Complications rates range from 18% to 45% in recent literature with a relatively large number of cases (**Table 1**).[2–6] In these reports, several factors associated with SSI were indicated: tumor location, advanced tumor stage, flap reconstruction, preoperative anemia, blood transfusion, operation times, tracheostomy, and others. On the other hand, previous irradiation and chemotherapy, and their effect on postoperative SSI, are still controversial.[5,7] These results are explained by the fact that most reports included a wide range of resection areas, varying previous treatments, various preoperative general conditions, and the possibility that outcome of reconstruction may be more technique-sensitive in patients with complicated defects and preoperative irradiation.

RETROSPECTIVE STUDIES CONCERNING WOUND COMPLICATIONS IN MICROVASCULAR TONGUE RECONSTRUCTION

In the past, the authors reviewed postoperative wound complications in 329 patients (240 men and 89 women; mean age, 56.0 years; age range, 20–87 years) who underwent microvascular tongue reconstruction after glossectomy for malignant tumors at the National Cancer Center Hospital from 1981 through 2002. Resection for primary tumors was performed in 210 patients, and for recurrent tumors in 119 patients. Previous irradiation had been performed in 92 patients. Partial glossectomy, oral hemiglossectomy, and hemiglossectomy involving half of the tongue had been performed in 121 patients, and subtotal or total glossectomy had been performed in 208 patients.

Several kinds of free flaps were primarily transferred: rectus abdominis musculocutaneous flaps in 231 patients, anterolateral thigh flaps in 47 patients, radial forearm flaps in 30 patients, and other

types of flaps in 21 patients. Postoperative significant wound complications were reviewed from the patient medical records.

Two hundred seventy-seven flaps survived perfectly; 36 (10.9%) survived with partial necrosis, and 16 (4.9%) underwent total necrosis. Significant local complications were not recognized in 184 patients (55.9%). Orocutaneous fistulas including total necrosis of the transferred flap developed in 73 patients (22.2%). Among them, major fistulas that required additional surgical treatment developed in 28 patients (8.5%). Patients with total necrosis of the free flap were included in the major fistula group. Abscesses were recognized in 145 patients (44.1%), and hematomas were recognized in 11 (3.3%) patients. These data on complications are shown in **Fig. 1**. **Fig. 2** shows the required wound-healing time from the first operation both in the group of abscesses without fistulas (70 patients) and in the group of fistulas (67 patients). Eight patients with abscesses were excluded because of local tumor recurrence. The median healing time of the abscess group was 25.5 days (9–155 days) and that of the fistula group was 36.0 days (9–730 days). Even though the patients' data included the dawn of microsurgical reconstruction at the head and neck region in Japan, these results indicated a high rate of SSI of microsurgical tongue reconstruction. The important finding was that abscesses and fistulas needed longer periods for wound healing and that this deteriorated the patient's general condition and reduced the quality of life by delaying recovery. SSI also increased the length of hospital stay, resulting in high medical costs.

Fig. 3 shows the overall survival rates for 325 cases of tongue cancer at the National Cancer Center Hospital in Japan in 2004. Generally, hemiglossectomy, subtotal, and total glossectomy patients need microsurgical reconstruction. The 5-year survival rate after total or subtotal glossectomy for tongue tumors is less than 40%; this means that half of the patients die within a year.

Table 1
The rate of surgical site infection in head and neck cancer surgeries

Authors, Year	Study Design	No. of Patients	Character of Disease	SSI Rate (%)
Penel et al,[2] 2005	Prospective	260	HN cancers	45.0
Liu et al,[3] 2007	Retrospective	1693	HN cancers	19.8
Karakida et al,[4] 2010	Retrospective	276	Free-flap HN cases	40.6
Lee et al,[5] 2011	Retrospective	697	HN cancers	18.4
Lin et al,[6] 2012	Retrospective	894	HN cancers	20.8

Abbreviation: HN, head and neck.

Wound Complications	No. of patients
No significant local complications	184 (55.9%)
Abscess formation	145 (44.1%)
Major orocutaneous fistula	28 (8.5%)
Minor orocutaneous fistula	45 (13.7%)
Hematoma	11 (3.3%)
Total flap necrosis	16 (4.9%)
Partial flap necrosis	36 (10.9%)

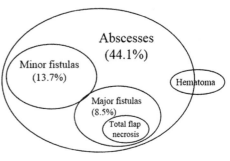

Relationship among the postoperative complications

Fig. 1. Wound complications during microsurgical tongue reconstruction at the National Cancer Center Hospital in Japan.

Therefore, SSI disrupted patients' lives, which were already shortened by the presence of the aggressive tumors.

Fig. 4 shows a representative unfavorable result case. The patient underwent resection of recurrent oral cancer and reconstruction with a free flap. Unfortunately, on the third postoperative day, an orocutaneous fistula developed and caused arterial thrombosis. Immediate salvage surgery was performed with a pectoralis major myocutaneous pedicled flap to cover the defect and the carotid artery. However, the peripheral part of the flap underwent necrosis, and a deltopectoral flap was transferred. After 8 additional operations, local recurrence was observed, and the patient died 10 months after the first reconstructive surgery.

EFFECT OF WOUND IRRADIATION ON SURGICAL SITE INFECTION

In general, the effect of radiotherapy on tissues can be divided into 2 phases: acute and chronic. In the acute phase, radiotherapy causes an inflammatory change in the skin, such as swelling and redness. The chronic phase of radiotherapy causes irreversible tissue degeneration. Vascular and perivascular changes lead to hypovascularity, tissue hypoxia, and eventually result in tissue fibrosis, skin atrophy, and intractable ulcers. Therefore, the discussion should be focused on the chronic phase of radiotherapy that may adversely affect wound healing. The study by Paydarfar and Birkmeyer[8] was limited to a review of pharyngocutaneous fistulas after total laryngectomy. This significant meta-analysis identified that preoperative radiotherapy and preoperative radiotherapy with concurrent neck dissection are the major risk factors for postoperative fistulas, while as described earlier, the adverse influence of a history of irradiation for postoperative SSI was controversial. However, if postoperative abscess formation or fistulas was noted, the time required for healing was longer in irradiated wounds than in nonirradiated wounds. These results indicate compromised wound healing in irradiated wounds.[7,9,10]

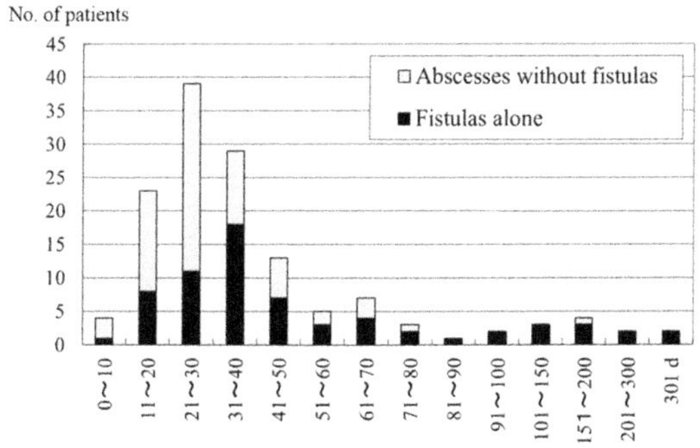

Fig. 2. Wound healing time both in the group of abscesses without fistulas and in the group of fistulas alone.

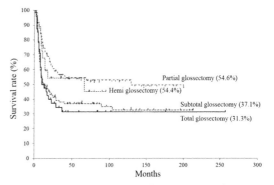

Fig. 3. Overall survival rates for 325 cases of tongue cancer in Japan. Parentheses indicate 5-year survival according to the type of tongue resection.

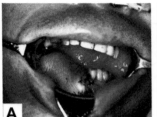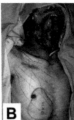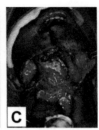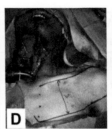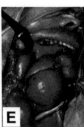

Fig. 4. An unfavorable result case following intraoral reconstruction. (*A*) Free rectus abdominis flap reconstruction for recurrent oral tumor. (*B*) On the third postoperative day, an orocutaneous fistula developed because of total necrosis of the flap. Immediate salvage surgery was performed with a pectoralis major myocutaneous pedicled flap. (*C*) The peripheral part of the flap underwent necrosis. (*D*) A deltopectoral flap was transferred to cover the carotid artery. (*E*) Wound condition after 8 additional surgeries. Local recurrence was recognized, and the patient died 10 months after the first reconstructive surgery.

Other problems with regard to irradiated wounds include poor inflammatory response to local complications that prevent the early identification and treatment of abscesses and fistulas, finally leading to major complications that require additional salvage operations.

To investigate the poor inflammatory reaction of the wound in the chronic phase, the authors reviewed 13 pharyngeal reconstruction cases with postoperative complications, such as local abscess formation, minor/major fistulas, and necrosis of the transferred flap at Okayama University Hospital from 2009 to 2012. In all patients, complications were noted after 5 postoperative days. **Table 2** shows the characteristics of patients and complications. Thirteen patients were classified into 3 groups. Patients in group A did not undergo irradiation and chemotherapy. Those in group B underwent neoadjuvant chemotherapy alone, and those in group C were in the chronic phase after irradiation. All patients in group C underwent salvage surgery for recurrent tumors. White blood cell (WBC) counts and C-reactive protein (CRP) levels were investigated retrospectively. **Fig. 5** shows the results of the postoperative changes of WBC counts and CRP levels. In group A, WBC counts fluctuated until 4 days after surgery. After 4 days, several peaks were noted due

---

Table 2
Characteristics of 13 patients and the distribution of groups A, B, and C with postoperative complications following head and neck cancer surgeries

Sex	12 M, 1 F
Mean age (range)	68.4 (51–85 y)
Tumor site (recurrence)	Lower gingiva: 1 (1) Laryngeal cancer: 4 (2) Oropharynx: 1 (0) Lower pharynx: 5 (2) Cervical pharynx: 2 (0)
Reconstructive methods	Primary closure: 1 Pectoralis major myocutaneous flap (PMMC): 4 Free jejunal graft: 6 Free jejunal graft + PMMC: 1 Free jejunal graft + Deltopectoral flap: 1

Group distribution and postoperative local complications (PC)
   Group A (5 patients): Preirradiation (−), neoajuvant chemotherapy (−)
     PC: Total flap necrosis 3, fistula 3, abscess without fistula 1
   Group B (3 patients): Preirradiation (−), neoajuvant chemotherapy (+)
     PC: Fistula 2, abscess without fistula 1
   Group C (5 patients): preirradiation (+)
     All patients underwent salvage surgery for recurrent tumor.
     Interval between Radiotherapy or chemoradiotherapy and operation; 31.6 mo (6–120 mo)
     PC: Total flap necrosis 1, fistula 2, abscess without fistula 2

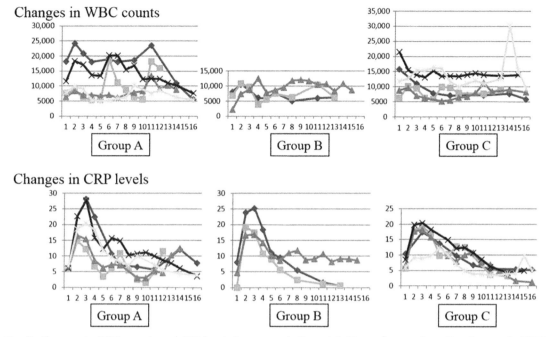

Fig. 5. Changes in WBC counts and CRP levels in groups A, B, and C. Upper figures show the changes in WBC counts, and lower figures show the changes in CRP levels. The longitudinal axis indicates the WBC counts and CRP levels; the horizontal axis indicates postoperative days.

to local complications. However, in groups B and C, the changes were very poor with the exception of one patient. As for CRP levels, until 5 days after surgery, they fluctuated in all groups. After 5 days, several peaks were noted in group A; however, the changes in groups B and C were subtle. Despite the fact that the sample size was small and a prospective study would have been more ideal, these results indicated a poor response to local infection in patients receiving chemotherapy or radiotherapy.

Fig. 6 shows a representative case of poor response to a local wound complication. The patient underwent salvage surgery after chemoradiotherapy with a free jejunal graft. Unfortunately, a fistula developed 6 days after surgery, and total necrosis was observed 7 days after surgery. Changes in WBC counts and CRP levels were

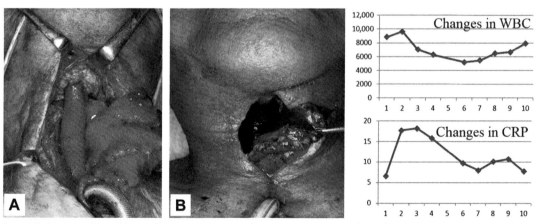

Fig. 6. (*left*) An unfavorable result case with poor inflammatory response. (*A*) A free jejunal graft was performed for salvage operation after chemoradiotherapy. (*B*) A major fistula was recognized 6 days postoperatively. (*right*) Changes in WBC counts and CRP levels.

minor. A poor reaction to the infection led to a delay in the detection of local complications.

STRATEGIES TO AVOID UNFAVORABLE RESULTS

There are many intraoperative conditions that contribute to unfavorable results (**Box 1**). In this section, the authors describe several significant intraoperative management strategies for avoiding unfavorable results.

Checking Blood Circulation in Transferred Flaps and Residual Tissues

Transferring or retaining tissues with unreliable blood circulation around defects must be avoided; this is because tissue defects requiring reconstruction in the head and neck area may already have been contaminated during surgery. To determine a reliable area for a transferred flap, the authors always use an indocyanine green fluorescence imaging with an infrared camera system (Photodynamic Eye; Hamamatsu Photonics, Hamamatsu, Japan). The authors took care of the circulation of the residual tissues, and if it is poor, they recommend that it should be removed during surgery. Partial necrosis of the mucosa, neck skin after irradiation, and thyroid tissue are often postoperatively seen.

Gentle Treatment and Suturing of the Wound

Marginal necrosis of the wound is often observed. Therefore, the authors want to emphasize the use of gentle suturing. They recommend that the ratio

---

Box 1
Considerable intraoperative conditions that contribute to the unfavorable result

1. Long operation time (bleeding, prolonged anesthesia)
2. Transfer unreliable tissues
3. Unreliable residual tissues (mucosa)
4. Choice of unreliable recipient vessels
5. Prolonged ischemic time of transferred tissues
6. Suture causing tissue ischemia
7. Dead space
8. Selection of the braided suture
9. Unsuitable selection and location of the drains
10. Insufficient hemostasis
11. Other

---

of the pitch to the bite be set at 2 or more, for maintaining blood circulation to the irradiated tissue (**Fig. 7**).

Management of the Dead Space

The most important point for avoiding unfavorable results is the management of dead space. Dead space is usually detected around the bone and artificial materials. Nonirradiated flexible skin can enter the dead space after surgery. However, irradiated skin cannot cover the dead space because of its hardness and lack of extensibility that requires much time for healing (**Fig. 8**). Attention should always be paid to the sufficient filling of the dead space using several portions of free flaps and pedicle flaps (**Fig. 9**).

Postoperatively, the transferred tissue is sometimes displaced from the grafted area and causes a new dead space. To avoid displacement of the flap, several anchoring sutures and the use of suction drainage are recommended. When the bone was resected, holes were created in the residual bone, and flaps were fixed to the bone through these holes using sutures (**Fig. 10**).

Selection of Recipient Vessels for Free Flap Transfer

To expose recipient vessels for free flap reconstruction in the previously operated and/or irradiated neck is extremely difficult. In 2009, Hanasono and colleagues[11] suggested an algorithm for locating recipient arteries and veins in irradiated wounds. The authors agree with that concept and take into consideration the advantages and disadvantages of the various techniques for finding alternative recipient vessels when the ipsilateral external carotid artery system and internal and external jugular venous systems are unavailable.

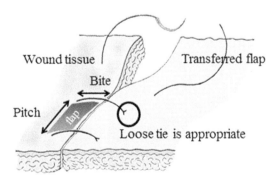

Fig. 7. Gentle treatment and suturing of the wound. The skin or mucosa area surrounded by the bite and pitch of the suture is one of the flaps. The ratio of the pitch to the bite is 2 or more.

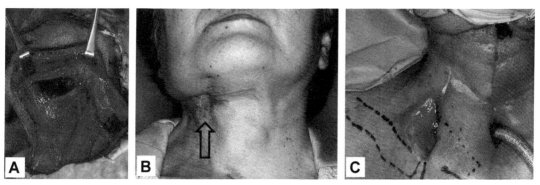

Fig. 8. Dead space around the defect. (*A*) Dead space is usually detected around the bone and artificial materials. (*B*) Nonirradiated flexible skin can enter the dead space (*arrow*) after surgery. (*C*) Irradiated skin cannot cover the dead space.

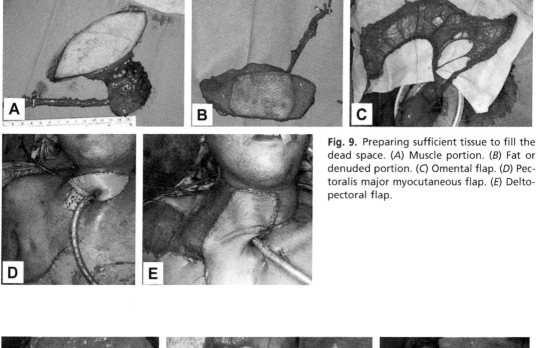

Fig. 9. Preparing sufficient tissue to fill the dead space. (*A*) Muscle portion. (*B*) Fat or denuded portion. (*C*) Omental flap. (*D*) Pectoralis major myocutaneous flap. (*E*) Deltopectoral flap.

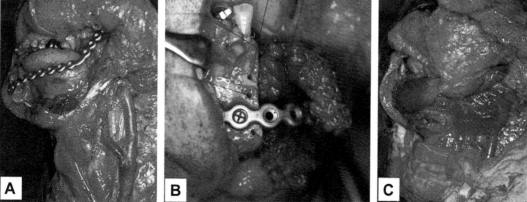

Fig. 10. Flap fixation to the residual bone. (*A*) A large dead space after hemimandibulectomy. (*B*) A transferred rectus abdominis musculocutaneous flap was fixed to the residual bone and reconstruction plate. (*C*) The dead space was fully filled with the flap.

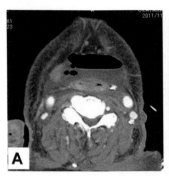
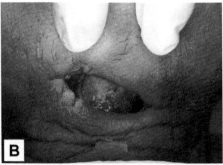
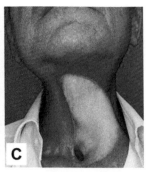

Fig. 11. CT examination 1 week after surgery in an irradiated patient. (*A*) CT image shows a large dead space and fluid pooling in the patient who underwent salvage surgery with a free jejunal graft. (*B*) Large dead space under the metal region. (*C*) After irrigation, a pectoralis major myocutaneous flap was transferred for filling the defect.

Careful Wound Check After Surgery

To avoid the progression of local complications, careful wound checks are necessary. If something is wrong, the wound should be immediately opened. In previously irradiated patients in particular, the authors sometimes missed the existence of SSI because of the poor inflammatory response of the wound. From their experience with these patients, severe local pain is a major symptom of a local infection.

In irradiated patients, the authors routinely use computed tomographic (CT) examinations to detect the dead space and fluid or air pooling 1 week after surgery. If a large dead space is detected, they open and irrigate the wound and consider additional surgery (**Fig. 11**).

Selection of the Appropriate Method for Salvaging Unfavorable Results

If an initial free flap undergoes total necrosis, the authors recommend a second free flap. In the past, they compared the healing time between conventional methods and free flaps as a salvage procedure, and they suggest that free flaps are an appropriate method for shortening the time of wound healing and hospitalization.[12] However, for transferring a second free flap, the appropriate management of early postoperative complications is essential. In other words, the early diagnosis of local complications, accurate assessment of wound conditions, and appropriate treatment of major fistulas are important.

Using these strategies for avoiding unfavorable results, the authors have recently reduced the rate of abscess and fistula formation.

SUMMARY

The authors suggest that local complications are inevitable in patients undergoing reconstruction in areas involving the head and neck. However, the frequency of major complications can be decreased, and late postoperative complications can be prevented using several appropriate methods.

REFERENCES

1. Mangram AJ, Horan TC, Pearson ML, et al. Guideline for prevention of surgical site infection, 1999. Hospital Infection Control Practices Advisory Committee. Infect Control Hosp Epidemiol 1999;20: 250–78.
2. Penel N, Fournier C, Lefebvre D, et al. Multivariate analysis of risk factors for wound infection in head and neck squamous cell carcinoma surgery with opening of mucosa. Study of 260 surgical procedures. Oral Oncol 2005;41:294–303.
3. Liu SA, Wong YK, Poon CK, et al. Risk factors for wound infection after surgery in primary oral cavity cancer patients. Laryngoscope 2007;117:166–71.
4. Karakida K, Aoki T, Ota Y, et al. Analysis of risk factors for surgical-site infections in 276 oral cancer surgeries with microvascular free-flap reconstructions at a single university hospital. J Infect Chemother 2010;16:334–9.
5. Lee DH, Kim SY, Nam SY, et al. Risk factors of surgical site infection in patients undergoing major oncological surgery for head and neck cancer. Oral Oncol 2011;47:528–31.
6. Lin WJ, Wang CP, Wang CC, et al. The association between surgical site infection and previous operation in oral cavity cancer patients. Eur Arch Otorhinolaryngol 2012;269:989–97.
7. Sugiyama N, Kimata Y, Sekido M, et al. A multi-institutional study of reconstruction for laryngopharyngoesophagectomy. Jpn J Head Neck Cancer 2006; 32:486–93.
8. Paydarfar JA, Birkmeyer NJ. Complications in head and neck surgery. Arch Otolaryngol Head Neck Surg 2006;132:67–72.

9. Virtaniemi JA, Kumpulainen EJ, Hirvikoski PP, et al. The incidence and etiology of postlaryngectomy pharyngocutaneous fistulae. Head Neck 2001;23: 29–33.

10. Chang DW, Hussussian C, Lewin JS, et al. Analysis of pharyngocutaneous fistula following free jejunal transfer for total laryngopharyngectomy. Plast Reconstr Surg 2002;109:1522–7.

11. Hanasono MM, Barnea Y, Skoracki RJ. Microvascular surgery in the previously operated and irradiated neck. Microsurgery 2009;29:1–7.

12. Onoda S, Kimata Y, Sugiyama N, et al. Secondary head and neck reconstruction using free flap to improve the postoperative function or appearance of cancer survivors. Microsurgery 2014;34: 122–8.

Fistulae After Successful Free Tissue Transfer to Head and Neck
Its Prevention and Treatment

 CrossMark

Nidal Farhan AL Deek, MSc, MD, Fu-Chan Wei, MD*,
Chung-Kan Tsao, MD

KEYWORDS

- Fistulas • Microsurgical head and neck reconstruction • Cancer • Radiotherapy • Free flap

KEY POINTS

- Oronasal and orocutaneous fistulae are among the untoward results of reconstructive microsurgery in head and neck cancer in spite of free flap viability.
- Complete obliteration of ablation-related dead spaces, adequate volume replacement, and water-tight closure of oral wounds ensure uneventful healing and prevent fistulae.
- Management of fistula ideally should not delay radiotherapy. However, reconstruction is timed based on wound condition, with consideration not to interrupt oncologic treatment.
- A second free flap may become necessary for the treatment of fistulae.

INTRODUCTION

Orocutaneous or oronasal fistula following microsurgical head and neck reconstruction is a bothersome complication that downgrades patient's quality of life and may jeopardize timely postoperative chemotherapy and radiotherapy administration.[1]

In literature, the reported incidence of fistulae has been as high as 20%, and a large percentage of fistulas received major second operation to achieve wound healing.[2–4] Reports dedicated to the causes of fistula, however, remain sparse and not comprehensive. Aside from the well-known patient-related risk factors such as poor nutritional status, systemic conditions that compromise wound healing, and radiotherapy and chemotherapy, knowledge on additional risk factors has been limited, in particular, the role of mistake in reconstructive surgery.

Furthermore, a systematic approach to head and neck fistulae after free flap reconstruction remains largely lacking. Wide-array of techniques such as vacuum-assisted closure,[5] local and regional flaps,[6,7] and free flaps[8] in addition to medical treatment[9] have been described but subjectively. The dilemma of deciding the optimal time for intervention with regards to adjuvant therapy administration and the optimal reconstructive option continues to confuse surgeons when confronted with a fistula.

Herein, this article will analyze fistulae from the perspective of poor planning, wrong design, and faulty execution of the surgery, and shares a simplified approach towards their management.

POOR PLANNING, IN VARIOUS DEFECTS

Poor planning can increase the risk of fistula, in particular, when the surgical plan results in

Conflict of Interest: The authors have no conflict of interest to declare.
Department of Plastic and Reconstructive Surgery, Chang Gung Memorial Hospital, Chang Gung Medical College, Chang Gung University, 199 Tun-Hwa North Road, Taipei 10591, Taiwan
* Correspondence author.
E-mail address: fuchanwei@gmail.com

Clin Plastic Surg 43 (2016) 739–745
http://dx.doi.org/10.1016/j.cps.2016.05.010
0094-1298/16/$ – see front matter © 2016 Elsevier Inc. All rights reserved.

improper flap selection to fulfill the reconstruction goal(s). The most common scenarios encountered include

- Anterior mandibular defect with associated substantial glossectomy defect when a soft tissue flap and reconstruction plate is planned (**Fig. 1**)[3]
- A composite or extensive composite mandibular defect, LC or LCL type based on the Jewer and Boyd classification, when a soft tissue flap and reconstruction plate are chosen (**Fig. 2**)[10]
- A high-volume maxillary defect when a bone flap is used[11]

Ideally, the first 2 scenarios should be reconstructed with double free flaps, a vascularized bone flap for segmental bone defect and soft tissue flap for dead space obliteration, soft tissue replacement, or coverage reconstruction (**Fig. 3**).[3,12] This option is associated with significantly fewer complications compared with the soft tissue flap and reconstruction plate option. On the other hand, the third scenario is better reconstructed with soft tissue flap to obliterate the dead space followed by bony reconstruction in a second stage.[13]

Defective planning leading to fistula can also include failure to identify and obliterate potential dead spaces after ablation surgeries. Such dead spaces may necessitate additional tissue components, larger skin paddle, particular inset techniques, or even a second free flap. Neglecting those inapt designs or faulty executions of reconstruction may lead to fistulae complication.[4]

In the commonly encountered glossectomy and mouth floor defects, the dead space following the resection of extrinsic tongue muscles needs to be obliterated adequately, not only to prevent fistulization, but also to support the neotongue for better function. It is worth noting that a deliberate suboptimal reconstructive plan is necessary sometime.

As stated in another article (see Nidal Farhan AL Deek, Fu-Chan Wei, and Huang-Kai Kao's article, "Free Tissue Transfer to Head and Neck: Lessons Learned from the Unfavorable Results—Experience per Subsite," in this issue), the surgeon may need to compromise by adopting a staged reconstruction with a free flap for the purpose of wound coverage only. This staged approach is deliberately chosen with complete awareness of possible tradeoffs such as fistula and other complications due to poor prognosis of the case. The situation is usually encountered in massive composite defects after ablation of recurrent or advanced secondary and tertiary tumors that otherwise should be reconstructed by double free flaps. The decision making, therefore, should always be guided by sound risk–benefit approach.

INAPT DESIGN

Given that the proper flaps have been chosen, design remains essential to fulfill the reconstructive goals. Dead space obliteration is 1 of these key goals; when not adequately fulfilled it may become a major risk factor for complications, including fistula. The flap, therefore, should be properly designed, ideally by an experienced surgeon to bring a reliable, suitably sized muscle or dermoadipofascial part of the skin paddle to achieve the goal.[14,15] The dead space between the hyoid bone and the mandible originally occupied by extrinsic tongue muscles can be a good example to illustrate the importance of good flap design. This space is usually about 5 × 3 × 3 cm in volume, and a reliable muscle segment can be included to fill the defect without compromising the viability of the rest of the flap and tongue reconstruction. A composite design of the myocutaneous flap, even made bigger than needed, may not be able to reconstruct the tongue and obliterate the dead space at the same time, while a

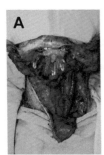 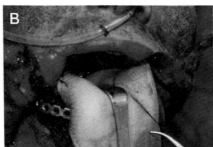 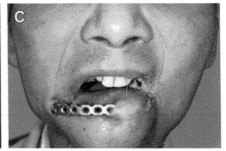

Fig. 1. (*A*) The defect after resection involving the total tongue, total lower lip, right segmental mandibulectomy from left body to right angle, left marginal mandibulectomy, and left inferior maxillectomy. (*B*) In flap inset, the skin was brought on top of the plate, while the muscle was underneath it to obliterate dead space. (*C*) Plate exposure after radiotherapy.

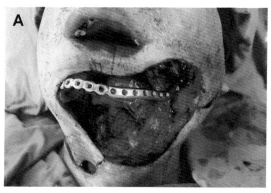
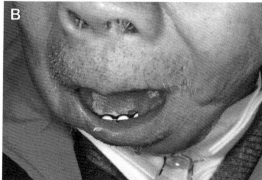

Fig. 2. (*A*) Composite segmental mandibulectomy with partial glossectomy after tumor resection. (*B*) Plate exposure intraorally after radiotherapy.

combined flap design could be more reliable in achieving this goal (**Fig. 4**).

The authors believe that for mouth floor reconstruction, complete obliteration with suitable tissue bulk is important to avoid fistula at the mouth floor or dropped, sunken, mouth floor.

CASE STUDY

This case involves a 73 year-old woman diagnosed with $T_2N_0M_0$ squamous cell carcinoma of the right tongue. She received hemiglossectomy and mouth floor resection. She developed orocutaneous fistula at the chin caused by inadequate obliteration of dead space at mouth floor. Fistula was managed conservatively until radiotherapy was completed; she then received subsequent free flap (**Fig. 5**).

Flap design becomes important when the patient has a past history of or is going to receive radiotherapy, which is a predisposing factor for fistula, due to tissue atrophy, scarring, contracture, and poor circulation.[16] Herein, the actual defect

is almost always bigger than the anticipated one, and the flap should always be made larger to allow tension-free closure.

ERRONEOUS EXECUTION OF THE RECONSTRUCTION

Failure to perform flawless reconstruction in spite of having proper planning and flap design could still lead to fistula, either immediately postoperatively, or after radiotherapy. Flawless execution that avoids fistula should ensure total obliteration of the dead space with viable tissue, as nonviable tissue becomes necrotic, inviting infection and resulting in fistula. The part of the flap stuffed in the dead space should be checked for reliability after establishing perfusion, especially when excess muscle is trimmed or its orientation is changed during inset of the flap. Flawless execution should also address all fibrotic and in-doubt tissue left after ablation surgery, especially if the patient has a history of irradiation or proven osteoradionecrosis.[17] Leaving borderline tissue

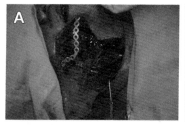
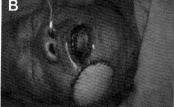
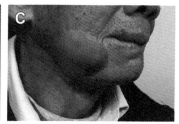
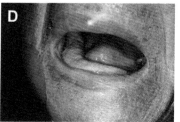

Fig. 3. (*A*) The defect after tumor resection, which was composite segmental mandibulectomy from right parasymphesis to right subcondyle, with reconstruction plate, in 2006. (*B*) Appearance at the end of reconstructive surgery; the osteoseptocutaneous fibula flap was used for bone and mouth floor reconstruction, while the anterolateral thigh flap was used for lining, skin, and volume augmentation. (*C, D*) Appearance after reconstruction with good volume restoration and contour, in 2009.

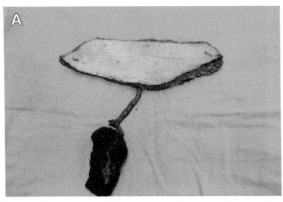
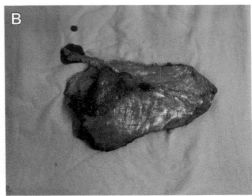

Fig. 4. (*A*) A segment of vastus lateralis muscle included in the harvested anterolateral thigh flap in a combined flap design. (*B*) A segmental of vastus lateralis muscle included in the harvested anterolateral thigh flap in a compound flap design.

may lead to dehiscence and fistula. Similarly, the bone after combined mandibulotomy and marginal mandibulectomy may not be healthy.[18] Conversion segmental mandibulectomy and total change in the reconstruction plan into vascularized bone flap instead of soft tissue flap could be needed to avoid complications.

Another aspect of impeccable execution is water-tight closure, in particular, for floor of the mouth and lip-alveolar sulcus repair, as they are dependent parts for saliva accumulation. Meticulous, multilayer, and mattress sutures can distribute tension to minimize tear of the suture line, dehiscence, and fistula. As the flap is usually tougher than the replaced or its adjacent tissues, it is better to work more on the flap side to avoid tearing the fragile gingiva.

The reconstruction plate, in combination with either bone or soft tissue flap, deserves special attention during flap inset to avoid complications.

Reconstruction Plate with Vascularized Bone

In this scenario, a major gap between the plate and bone could be a potential problem. Increasing the number of osteotomies may minimize that gap; however, in some cases, it may come at the price of compromising bone viability. Based on the authors' review of 80 recent cases of mandibular reconstruction with the MatrixMandible (Synthes, West Chester, PA) preformed plate, a gap between the bone and plate is allowed to some degree, given that the space between the plate and bone is filled by a soft tissue component of an osteocutaneous flap, like the soleus muscle, while the plate and the bone are also covered by reliable tissue such as from another part of the compound flap, an oversized skin paddle draped over them (**Fig. 6**).

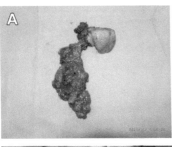
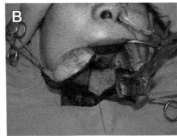
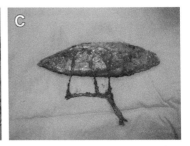
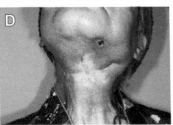
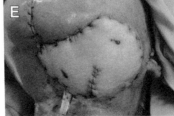

Fig. 5. (*A*) The excised hemitongue with mouth floor and lymph nodes levels I-III. (*B*) The defect after resection. (*C*) The anterolateral thigh flap based on 3 myocutaneous perforators in 2013. (*D*) The orocutaneous fistula at the submandibular area in 2014. (*E*) The second anteroalateral thigh flap in place in 2014.

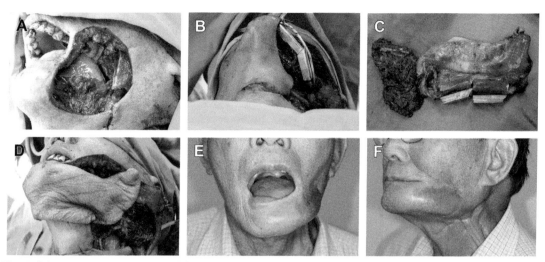

Fig. 6. (*A*) Extensive composite mandibular defect after cancer excison. (*B*) Gap and dead space between reconstruction plate and vascularized fibula. (*C*) An osteotomized fibula osteoseptocutaneous flap including large skin paddle and a soleus muscle. (*D*) Inset of the flap. (*E*, *F*) One-year postoperative follow-up.

Reconstruction Plate and Soft Tissue Flap

In this scenario, the lack of adequate tissue around the plate or tissue atrophy after radiotherapy could be a potential problem. For these cases, a musculocutaneous flap instead of cutaneous flap only could be a better choice, as it allows the plate to be completely wrapped with the muscle component,[19] preferably, bringing the suture line inferior to the plate, not on top of it, to prevent dehiscence due to gravity and muscle weight (**Fig. 7**).

A SIMPLIFIED APPROACH TO OROCUTANEOUS AND ORONASOCUTANEOUS FISTULA

Microsurgical head and neck reconstruction is a major surgery and aims at providing full and timely wound healing and achieving optimal functional and aesthetic results.

The nasoorocutaneous fistula threatens these goals. The patient becomes anxious to leave the hospital early, to know what needs to be done, and how long it is going to take until full recovery. The surgeon needs to answer these questions with an eye on the calendar if chemotherapy and radiotherapy are expected, and many times is confused with selection of the optimal technique(s).

Based on the presentation of the fistula, a new useful approach can be employed.

When the flap is not at risk of compromised viability, the wound is not infected, and the fistula has no large output, a less-aggressive but effective management can be done with vacuum-assisted closure (VAC).[5]

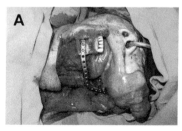
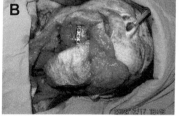
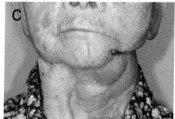
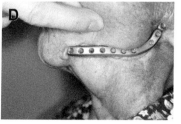

Fig. 7. (*A*) The preformed reconstruction plate in place after tumor resection. (*B*) Flap inset; the muscle was wrapped around the plate while the skin was deepithelialized and brought on top of the plate to provide additional coverage and augment the cheek skin, replacing some of the missing bulk after resection. (*C*, *D*) In spite of plate exposure after radiotherapy, the patient had symmetric face without fistula in 2015; the plate then was removed uneventfully.

When conditions are not permissive for VAC, the patient should be sent back to the operation room for adequate debridement, if needed, flap inset adjustment, and adequate wound repair if there is dehiscence. If a large portion of the flap is debrided, and the wound cannot be closed, a second free flap or regional flap depending on prognosis, tissue quality, and fistula size should be planned within a week after the first debridement,[20] provided the wound remains clean. Waiting for some time before the reconstruction allows the surgeon a second look and complete elimination of in-doubt tissue/border line tissue from the first debridement.

If a neglected fistula is noted during the patient's return visit to the clinic and before radiotherapy, the authors prefer to discuss the case with the ablative and radiologist teams to decide the time schedule for radiotherapy and wound management.

When patients present with the fistulae while on radiotherapy, radiotherapy should not be interrupted,[21] and the fistula is managed conservatively by less aggressive but effective wound care until radiotherapy is completed and a definite reconstruction planned. When fistulae present right after radiotherapy, the wound is managed by adequate wound care to prevent infection and minimize fibrosis. Reassurance is important at this step, as the patient could be bothered by the wound condition, with pain and discomfort. It is better to wait for some time until the tissue settles and inflammation signs subside. The quality of tissue and the size of the fistula then determine the reconstructive course and options. Although the fistula can be successfully treated with local or regional tissue,[6,7] when there is no significant scarring around or the fistula is of small size, the authors' technique of choice is a well-planned second free flap in collaboration with a head and neck cancer ablation surgeon,[22–24] since many of these patients present not only with fistula, but also with other coexisting unfavorable conditions such as tissue atrophy, plate exposure, trismus, or even occult recurrence, which ideally can be addressed at the same time.

Honoring the goal of enhanced patient's quality of life will necessitate a broader view of the problem that is not limited to the fistula, and such view may only be fulfilled with a free flap. Another reason for the authors' preference is that regional flaps such as the deltopectoral and pectoralis major come with higher complication rates[6,25] and may eventually necessitate a salvage free flap.[20]

It is only when a second free flap is not possible that a regional flap is chosen. The flap of choice for that scenario remains the pectoralis major, resulting in upside down reconstructive ladder.[26]

CASE STUDY (2)

48-year-old man diagnosed with left mouth floor cancer T2N0M0 received wide resection and reconstruction with radial forearm flap. The patient developed orocutaneous fistula at the submandibular area in 2010. The patient received serial fistulectomies and debridements without definite cure. In 2014, the fistula was excised, and the wound was closed by means of free radial forearm flap. The fistula never relapsed since then (**Fig. 8**).

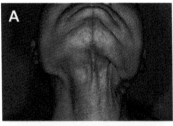
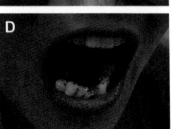
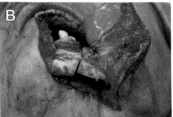
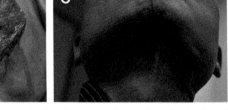

Fig. 8. (*A*) Persistent communication between the oral cavity and neck skin for 6 years. (*B*) Fistulectomy necessitating mandibulotomy. (*C, D*) Fistula closed, appearance 1 year after fistulectomy and a small forearm flap reconstruction.

SUMMARY

The incidence of fistula after head and neck cancer excision and microsurgical reconstruction could be reduced with optimization of the surgical plan, technique, and execution. It is more important to decide a guideline for management based on presentation and timing of radiotherapy over technique selection algorithms. Free flaps remain the authors' reliable reconstructive option in most cases of orocutaneous and nasocutaneous fistulae.

REFERENCES

1. Momeni A, Kim RY, Kattan A, et al. Microsurgical head and neck reconstruction after oncologic ablation: a study analyzing health-related quality of life. Ann Plast Surg 2013;70(4):462–9.

2. Hidalgo DA, Pusic AL. Free-flap mandibular reconstruction: a 10-year follow-up study. Plast Reconstr Surg 2002;110(2):438–49 [discussion: 450–1].

3. Miyamoto S, Sakuraba M, Nagamatsu S, et al. Comparison of reconstruction plate and double flap for reconstruction of an extensive mandibular defect. Microsurgery 2012;32(6):452–7.

4. Vega C, León X, Cervelli D, et al. Total or subtotal glossectomy with microsurgical reconstruction: functional and oncological results. Microsurgery 2011;31(7):517–23.

5. Andrews BT, Smith RB, Hoffman HT, et al. Orocutaneous and pharyngocutaneous fistula closure using a vacuum-assisted closure system. Ann Otol Rhinol Laryngol 2008;117(4):298–302.

6. Andrews BT, McCulloch TM, Funk GF, et al. Deltopectoral flap revisited in the microvascular era: a single-institution 10-year experience. Ann Otol Rhinol Laryngol 2006;115(1):35–40.

7. Rigby MH, Hayden RE. Regional flaps: a move to simpler reconstructive options in the head and neck. Curr Opin Otolaryngol Head Neck Surg 2014;22(5):401–6.

8. Ross G, Yla-Kotola TM, Goldstein D, et al. Second free flaps in head and neck reconstruction. J Plast Reconstr Aesthet Surg 2012;65(9):1165–8.

9. Ahn D, Sohn JH, Jeong JY. Chyle fistula after neck dissection: an 8-year, single-center, prospective study of incidence, clinical features, and treatment. Ann Surg Oncol 2015;22(Suppl 3):1000–6.

10. Wei FC, Celik N, Yang WG, et al. Complications after reconstruction by plate and soft-tissue free flap in composite mandibular defects and secondary salvage reconstruction with osteocutaneous flap. Plast Reconstr Surg 2003;112(1):37–42.

11. Hanasono MM, Silva AK, Yu P, et al. A comprehensive algorithm for oncologic maxillary reconstruction. Plast Reconstr Surg 2013;131(1):47–60.

12. Wei FC, Demirkan F, Chen HC, et al. Double free flaps in reconstruction of extensive composite mandibular defects in head and neck cancer. Plast Reconstr Surg 1999;103(1):39–47.

13. Cordeiro PG, Chen CM. A 15-year review of midface reconstruction after total and subtotal maxillectomy: part I. Algorithm and outcomes. Plast Reconstr Surg 2012;129(1):124–36.

14. Cordova A, D'Arpa S, Di Lorenzo S, et al. Prophylactic chimera anterolateral thigh/vastus lateralis flap: preventing complications in high-risk head and neck reconstruction. J Oral Maxillofac Surg 2014; 72(5):1013–22.

15. Girod DA, McCulloch TM, Tsue TT, et al. Risk factors for complications in clean-contaminated head and neck surgical procedures. Head Neck 1995;17(1):7–13.

16. Celik N, Wei FC, Chen HC, et al. Osteoradionecrosis of the mandible after oromandibular cancer surgery. Plast Reconstr Surg 2002;109(6):1875–81.

17. Wang CC, Cheng MH, Hao SP, et al. Osteoradionecrosis with combined mandibulotomy and marginal mandibulectomy. Laryngoscope 2005;115(11):1963–7.

18. Fanzio PM, Chang KP, Chen HH, et al. Plate exposure after anterolateral thigh free-flap reconstruction in head and neck cancer patients with composite mandibular defects. Ann Surg Oncol 2015;22(9):3055–60.

19. Wei FC, Demirkan F, Chen HC, et al. The outcome of failed free flaps in head and neck and extremity reconstruction: what is next in the reconstructive ladder? Plast Reconstr Surg 2001;108(5):1154–60 [discussion: 1161–2].

20. Lau V, Chen LM, Farwell DG, et al. Postoperative radiation therapy for head and neck cancer in the setting of orocutaneous and pharyngocutaneous fistula. Am J Clin Oncol 2011;34(3):276–80.

21. Hao SP, Chen HC, Wei FC, et al. Systematic management of osteoradionecrosis in the head and neck. Laryngoscope 1999;109(8):1324–7 [discussion: 1327–8].

22. Chun JK, Senderoff DM. Microsurgical reconstruction of difficult orocutaneous fistulas. Ann Plast Surg 1996;36(4):417–24.

23. Hanasono MM, Corbitt CA, Yu P, et al. Success of sequential free flaps in head and neck reconstruction. J Plast Reconstr Aesthet Surg 2014;67(9): 1186–93.

24. Kekatpure VD, Trivedi NP, Manjula BV, et al. Pectoralis major flap for head and neck reconstruction in era of free flaps. Int J Oral Maxillofac Surg 2012; 41(4):453–7.

25. Lundgren TK, Wei FC. Oversized design of the anterolateral thigh flap for head and neck reconstruction. J Craniofac Surg 2013;24(1):134–5.

26. Mardini S, Wei FC, Salgado CJ, et al. Reconstruction of the reconstructive ladder. Plast Reconstr Surg 2005;115(7):2174.

Trismus Secondary Release Surgery and Microsurgical Free Flap Reconstruction After Surgical Treatment of Head and Neck Cancer

Yang-Ming Chang, DDS, Nidal Farhan AL Deek, MSc, MD,
Fu-Chan Wei, MD*

KEYWORDS

- Trismus • Free flap reconstruction • Coronoidectomy • Radial forearm flap
- One donor site two anterolateral thigh flaps

KEY POINTS

- Trismus is a significant untoward outcome after head and neck cancer-ablation reconstruction, even by a free flap whether or not radiotherapy has been delivered.
- The only effective way to correct the unfavorable course of trismus is adequate release and reconstruction with another free flap. Achieving durable results after trismus release and free flap reconstruction necessitates proper patient selection, patients compliance, and vigorous rehabilitation.

INTRODUCTION

Trismus is not uncommon after head and neck cancer ablation and reconstruction.[1,2] The combined effect of resection surgery that is destructive in its nature, radiotherapy, and preexisting limited mouth opening contributes to trismus.[3,4] In such a case, trismus can be considered as a disease entity that may benefit from secondary surgical release and reconstruction. Alternatively, trismus could be a sign of a serious illness such as osteoradionecrosis or secondary/recurrent tumor, and if that the case, surgery should target the underlying condition and may result in possible improvement of trismus.[5,6]

Trismus compromises patient quality of life due to its adverse effects on chewing, swallowing, articulation, and oral hygiene.[7] It also limits tumor surveillance, which could delay appropriate intervention.[8,9] Therefore, a surgical effort towards adequate release and proper reconstruction when indicated can have a significant positive impact on patient's satisfaction and facilitates tumor control.[10]

Favorable outcomes and long-standing results after trismus release surgery and reconstruction, however, are built on proper patient selection, meticulous but adequate multistructure release, and proper reconstruction techniques that can address additional patient's goals such as improved oral function, enhanced facial appearance and cosmesis, and dental rehabilitation.[4,10]

Herein, this article will focus on the conditions and factors essential for fulfilling the goals of trismus release and reconstruction surgeries and their possible pitfalls and their avoidance.

Department of Plastic and Reconstructive Surgery, Chang Gung Memorial Hospital, Chang Gung Medical College, Chang Gung University, 199 Tun-Hwa North Road, Taipei 10591, Taiwan
* Corresponding author.
E-mail address: fuchanwei@gmail.com

Clin Plastic Surg 43 (2016) 747–752
http://dx.doi.org/10.1016/j.cps.2016.06.002

PATIENT SELECTION AND PITFALLS

The importance of selection of the right candidate for release surgery and free flap reconstruction cannot be overemphasized. Motivated and compliant patients noted during postablation reconstruction follow-up are ideal.

Mouth opening and trismus history should be well documented, as they may help identify patients at risk of malignancy if trismus is sudden or to determine the benefits of surgery if trismus was an old finding before the initial resection–reconstruction.

Tempomandibular joints (TMJ) and cheek pliability are also carefully examined.

In preparation for surgery, panoramic pictures, pneumatic computed tomography (CT), and standard cancer survey are performed to rule out malignancy and provide means to assess functional gain.[4,11]

Pitfalls may occur including selection of those who may not benefit from the surgery at all, such as patients with TMJ and patients with extensive history of cancer resection, reconstruction, and postoperative radiotherapy.

Patients with TMJ ankylosis may increasingly experience relapse of ankylosis and gain no or limited mouth opening even after surgery. The authors largely have avoided those patients; however, in some selected cases, TMJ ankylosis could be addressed first, and then after achieving stable results, release surgery can follow.

SURGICAL RELEASE OF TRISMUS AND ITS PITFALLS

Trismus release can be achieved by variety of techniques.[12,13] Scar release followed by masticatory muscles myotomy and combined with coronoidotomy/coronoidectomy to diminish the locking effect of temporalis muscle fibers can yield good and lasting results.[14] This extensive, multistructure release requires a complete understanding of the multifactorial nature of trismus[3,4] to achieve the goals.

Although wound healing and contracture are individual, unpredictable, and inevitable, patient's compliance with rehabilitation may also count greatly for the ultimate result, and it could result in 50% loss of intraoperative gain in mouth opening on long term follow-up. However, in the authors' practice, repeated release surgery has never been indicated, suggesting that the long-term gain in mouth opening is enough and acceptable for the patients.

In contrast to inadequacy is excessive release surgery, resulting in bilateral tempomandibular joint dislocation. Avoidance demands unforceful release and to set the goal of mouth opening to not to exceed 40 to 45 mm. The release procedures should be individualized but always start from simple scar resection, all the way up to combined multistructure release including coronoidotomy based on intraoperative mouth opening gain after each step of release.

RECONSTRUCTION TECHNIQUES AND THEIR PITFALLS

After adequate release, optimal reconstruction is necessary to achieve long lasting gain in mouth opening.[4,10] Free flap is the method of choice, because it allows primary wound healing with minimal destruction to local/regional tissue, minimizing postoperative inflammation and contracture.

Proper free flap selection and inset are essential for uncomplicated reconstruction and maintenance of good results.

The Donor Site of Choice

In free flap selection, bulk and rigidity should be considered first. Bulky flaps will necessitate revision surgery, as they endanger self-chewing, resulting in prolonged inflammation, leading to tissue contracture and regression of the initially gained mouth opening. Therefore, they are better to be avoided.

In the search for the optimal thickness of the flap with minimal donor site morbidity to reconstruct the release defect, the authors' experience has focused on 2 donor sites, the radial forearm and the anterolateral thigh. This choice evolved from using

Bilateral radial forearm flaps, to 1 longer radial forearm flap to avoid bilateral loss of the radial artery

To two radial forearm flaps from the same donor site to avoid using the lip-gingival sulcus as a tunnel for 1 longer radial forearm flap damaging lower lip function

To bilateral anterolateral thigh flaps to allow simultaneous harvest and release

To 2 anterolateral thigh flaps from the same donor site as experience and familiarity with the anatomy improved

Into finally bilateral radial forearm flaps given negligible morbidity after sacrificing the radial artery based on experience with more than 1000 forearm flaps and reliability of anatomy compared with 2 radial forearm flaps from one side

To a lesser degree, 2 anterolateral thigh flaps from the same donor site are still selected in some patients who have relatively thin lateral thigh skin.

The radial forearm flap compared with the anterolateral thigh flap is thinner and more pliable. Although the anterolateral thigh (ALT) can be thinned,[15] it remains more rigid than the radial forearm flap,[16] and this rigidity may limit tissue stretchability, restricting mouth opening and oral cavity volume. Furthermore, the donor site of the radial forearm flap can be closed primarily if the intraoral defect after release is not wider than 2 to 3 cm (**Fig. 1**).

When trismus release surgery results in wider soft tissue loss, greater than 3 cm in width, or the surgery aims at volume augmentation to enhance appearance at the same operation, the anterolateral thigh flap is indicated. The flap can fulfill these goals, and the donor site can still be closed primarily.[17] The possibility of harvesting 2 ALTs from the same donor site based on 2 different skin vessels is well-established.[18]

Alternative Donor Sites

To achieve tumor ablation and release of trismus simultaneously, marginal mandibulectomy and segmental mandibulectomy could be indicated.

In some of these cases, the initial reconstruction can be a soft tissue flap with/without reconstruction plate, although it may have higher rate of plate exposure, fracture, malocclusion, trismsus, and even fistula[19] (**Fig. 2**).

The other option can be an osteocutaneous flap reconstruction aiming at dental rehabilitation as well (**Fig. 3**).

In the authors' experience, the vascularized osteoseptocutaneous fibula flap is an ideal choice under this consideration with minimal donor site morbidity. The skin paddle can be designed as a long and narrow ellipse to allow primary closure at the donor site if the need for intraoral lining or external skin is not wider than 3.5 cm.[20] Furthermore, even if a patient does not seek dental restoration, the additional bone height of the mandible flap bone graft provides skeletal support to resist recurrence of contracture.[21]

With optimization of free flap selection and avoidance of locoregional tissue, pitfalls in reconstruction still can occur, which are largely attributed to flap design and inset. It is important for this particular reconstruction not to have bulky flap bulging in between the molars to avoid the flap getting bitten or chewed; therefore, the flap should not be designed wider than the defect itself when the mouth is closed, but it should have the same length. The inset starts with suturing the tip of the flap to the most posterior wound at the

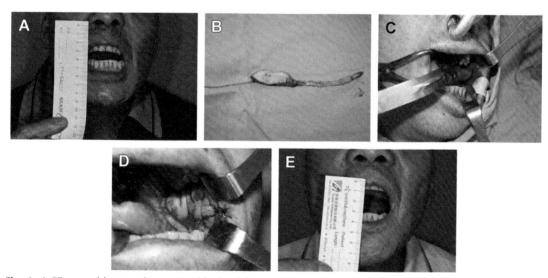

Fig. 1. A 57-year-old man who received leukoplakia excision and reconstruction with artificial dermis in 2003, then diagnosed with hypopharyngeal cancer in 2012 for which he received chemotherapy and radiotherapy presented with long-standing trismus with IID measured 12 mm. (*A*) At the initial consultation, trismus with 12 mm IID. (*B*) Bilateral radial forearm flaps 2.5 cm in width for reconstruction of mucosal defect after release. (*C*) The defect measured less than 3 cm in width after trismus release surgery. (*D*) Intraoperative appearance after reconstruction. (*E*) After 2-year of follow-up, postoperative gain in the mouth opening was 8 mm, and IID was 20 mm, in 2015.

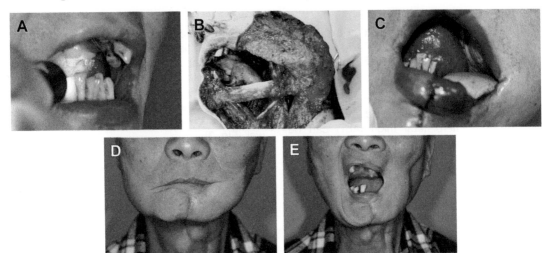

Fig. 2. A 49-year-old man diagnosed with left buccal squamous cell carcinoma (SCC) cancer T2N0M0 and trismus with 15 mm MMO presented for cancer ablation, trismus release, and reconstruction. (*A*) The buccal cancer and trismus with 15 mm MMO in 2014. (*B*) The defect after tumor resection involved inferior maxillectomy, marginal mandibulectomy, and left buccal region. (*C*) Appearance after adequate reconstruction with anterolateral thigh flap. (*D, E*) Appearance with good contour and 25 mm MMO mouth opening in 2016.

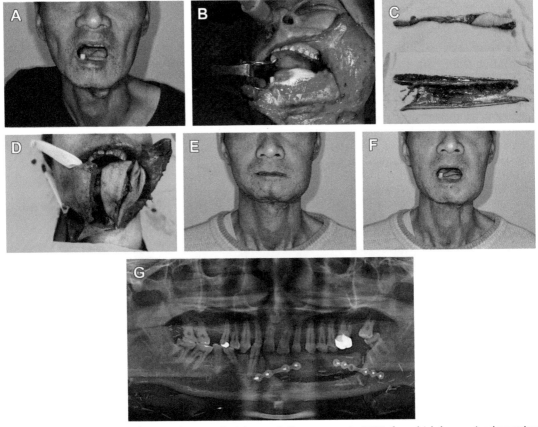

Fig. 3. A 48-year-old man who was diagnosed with mouth floor cancer in 2012, for which he received marginal mandibulectomy and ALT flap reconstruction presented with left-side submucosa fibrosis and right-sided buccal scar contracture, deficiency in mandible height, and sunken appearance. (*A*) Trismus and sunken lower face appearance in 2013. (*B*) The defects after adequate scar release. (*C*) The radial forearm flap and fibula osteoseptocutaneous flap used for reconstruction of both sides. (*D*) The fibula osteoseptocutaneous flap as an onlay graft to the remaining left mandible. (*E, F*) Appearance and mouth opening with adequate filling of the lower face in 2014. (*G*) Panorex of the mandible in 2014.

trigone and proceeds anteriorly with the flap pulled up at proper tension, then sutured in in-to-out manner.

POSTOPERATIVE FOLLOW-UP AND REHABILITATION

Close follow-up to check patient's compliance with rehabilitation is important. There is no superior exercise therapy over another.[12] Therefore, the authors do not recommend particular stretching exercises, certain duration or repetition; however, they do advise a readily available, economical, and patient-friendly method. Wooden tongue depressors placed between molars during rest and sleep are useful. Patients are encouraged to do both stretching and cheek-blowing exercises as frequently and as long as possible, especially in the first year after operation.

Maximal mouth opening (MMI) or inter-incisors distance (IID) should be measured regularly. Postoperative air contrast pneumatic CT is also performed too, at 6 months after surgery. The authors' results have shown improved maximal buccal vestibular volume and improvement in buccal mucosal elasticity.[11]

SUMMARY

Trismus is a life-debilitating condition that is best treated with surgical release and free flap reconstruction. Adequate release often necessitates scar release and masticatory muscles group myotomy combined with coronoidotomy. Proper free flap reconstruction and vigorous mouth opening exercises can yield long-lasting results. Optimizing patient selection, free flap inset, and avoidance of excessive and forceful release can eliminate the unfavorable results following this unique surgery.

REFERENCES

1. Pauli N, Johnson J, Finizia C, et al. The incidence of trismus and long-term impact on health-related quality of life in patients with head and neck cancer. Acta Oncol 2013;52(6):1137–45.
2. Hanasono MM, Corbitt CA, Yu P, et al. Success of sequential free flaps in head and neck reconstruction. J Plast Reconstr Aesthet Surg 2014;67(9): 1186–93.
3. Steiner F, Evans J, Marsh R, et al. Mouth opening and trismus in patients undergoing curative treatment for head and neck cancer. Int J Oral Maxillofac Surg 2015;44(3):292–6.
4. Mardini S, Chang YM, Tsai CY, et al. Release and free flap reconstruction for trismus that develops after previous intraoral reconstruction. Plast Reconstr Surg 2006;118(1):102–7.
5. Oh HK, Chambers MS, Martin JW, et al. Osteoradionecrosis of the mandible: treatment outcomes and factors influencing the progress of osteoradionecrosis. J Oral Maxillofac Surg 2009;67(7): 1378–86.
6. Rapidis AD, Dijkstra PU, Roodenburg JL, et al. Trismus in patients with head and neck cancer: etiopathogenesis, diagnosis and management. Clin Otolaryngol 2015;40(6):516–26.
7. Johnson J, Johansson M, Rydén A, et al. Impact of trismus on health-related quality of life and mental health. Head Neck 2015;37(11):1672–9.
8. Weber C, Dommerich S, Pau HW, et al. Limited mouth opening after primary therapy of head and neck cancer. Oral Maxillofac Surg 2010;14(3):169–73.
9. Bouman MA, Dijkstra PU, Reintsema H, et al. Surgery for extra-articular trismus: a systematic review. Br J Oral Maxillofac Surg 2016;54(3): 253–9.
10. Chan CL, Wei FC, Tsao CK, et al. Free flap reconstruction after surgical release of oral submucous fibrosis:long term maintenance and its clinical implications. J Plast Reconstr Aesthet Surg 2014; 67:344–9.
11. Chang CC, Ng SH, Lam WL, et al. Using pneumocomputerized tomography as a quantitative assessment of result in submucous fibrosis patients treated with surgical release and free flap reconstruction. J Craniofac Surg 2014;25(6):1943–6.
12. Kamstra JI, van Leeuwen M, Roodenburg JL, et al. Exercise therapy for trismus secondary to head and neck cancer: a systematic review. Head Neck 2016. [Epub ahead of print].
13. Melchers LJ, Van Weert E, Beurskens CH, et al. Exercise adherence in patients with trismus due to head and neck oncology: a qualitative study into the use of the Therabite. Int J Oral Maxillofac Surg 2009;38(9):947–54.
14. Chang YM, Tsai CY, Kildal M, et al. Importance of coronoidotomy and masticatory muscle myotomy in surgical release of trismus caused by submucous fibrosis. Plast Reconstr Surg 2004;113(7): 1949–54.
15. Sun G, Lu M, Hu Q, et al. Clinical application of thin anterolateral thigh flap in the reconstruction of intraoral defects. Oral Surg Oral Med Oral Pathol Oral Radiol 2013;115(2):185–91.
16. Hwang K, Kim H, Kim DJ. Thickness of skin and subcutaneous tissue of the free flap donor sites: a histologic study. Microsurgery 2016;36(1):54–8.
17. Lutz BS, Wei FC. Microsurgical workhorse flaps in head and neck reconstruction. Clin Plast Surg 2005;32(3):421–30, vii.
18. Huang JJ, Wallace C, Lin JY, et al. Two small flaps from one anterolateral thigh donor site for bilateral

buccal mucosa reconstruction after release of submucous fibrosis and/or contracture. J Plast Reconstr Aesthet Surg 2010;63(3):440–5.

19. Wei FC, Celik N, Yang WG, et al. Complications after reconstruction by plate and soft-tissue free flap in composite mandibular defects and secondary salvage reconstruction with osteocutaneous flap. Plast Reconstr Surg 2003;112(1):37–42.

20. Wallace CG, Chang YM, Tsai CY, et al. Harnessing the potential of the free fibula osteoseptocutaneous flap in mandible reconstruction. Plast Reconstr Surg 2010;125(1):305–14.

21. Baumann DP, Yu P, Hanasono MM, et al. Free flap reconstruction of osteoradionecrosis of the mandible: a 10-year review and defect classification. Head Neck 2011;33(6):800–7.

The Osteosarcoradio-necrosis as an Unfavorable Result Following Head and Neck Tumor Ablation and Microsurgical Reconstruction

Nidal Farhan AL Deek, MSc, MD, Fu-Chan Wei, MD*

KEYWORDS

- Osteoradionecrosis • Osteosarcoradionecrosis • Radiotherapy

KEY POINTS

- The soft tissue has a core role in the development and management of osteoradionecrosis, preferably called osteosarcoradionecrosis.
- Debridement and sequestrectomy may induce further destruction to the tissue already damaged by radiotherapy; it is better to be avoided.
- Necrosis is irreversible condition; once osteosarcoradionecrosis is diagnosed, only resection and reconstruction can provide decisive, cost-effective treatment.
- The reconstruction has a potential role to manipulate the postablative course, decreasing complications following radiotherapy.

INTRODUCTION

The osteoradionecrosis is commonly defined as bone necrosis following radiotherapy. The presence of chronic, nonhealing wound with bone necrosis for more than 3 months in the setting of previous radiotherapy and in the absence of tumor recurrence or metastasis is necessary for diagnosis.[1,2] Risk factors are well-identified and numerous and include the mandible, T3 and T4 tumors, alcohol and tobacco use, and radiotherapy dose of at least 60 Gy.[1,2] Three theories have been suggested since 1970 in an attempt to explain why and how osteoradionecrosis develops and progresses.[3–5] Although none of them is conclusive, Delanian's theory of radiation-induced fibroatrophy seems to have stronger evidence.[5,6] Classifications are plenty, and they all try to utilize different treatment modalities such as medical therapy, hyperbaric oxygen, debridement and sequestrectomy, and resection and flap reconstruction in a stepwise approach.[1,2,4,7–9]

However, scrutinizing what the literature has on osteoradionecrosis this far starting with the definition of osteoradionecrosis and ending up with treatment modalities, using logic, science, and experience to accept or reject findings bring to attention that osteoradionecrosis is not a

Conflict of Interest: The authors have no conflict of interest to declare.
Department of Plastic and Reconstructive Surgery, Chang Gung Memorial Hospital, Chang Gung University Medical College, Chang Gung University, Taipei, Taiwan
* Corresponding author. Department of Plastic and Reconstructive Surgery, Chang Gung Memorial Hospital, Chang Gung University Medical College, 199 Tun-Hwa North Road, Taipei 10591, Taiwan.
E-mail address: fuchanwei@gmail.com

Clin Plastic Surg 43 (2016) 753–759
http://dx.doi.org/10.1016/j.cps.2016.05.009
0094-1298/16/$ – see front matter © 2016 Elsevier Inc. All rights reserved.

bone-only disease entity. Mucositis, xerostomia, and soft tissue necrosis, fibrosis, and atrophy are all important features of osteoradionecrosis[10] that need not to be omitted from the definition or treatment plan. Furthermore, classifications, which in general aim at staging bone necrosis to guide therapy, may seem self-contradictory or illogical in the sense that necrosis is necrosis, which cannot be staged, but can be quantified, instead. This is particularly important, because if one agrees with the fact that necrosis is death of the tissue, an irreversible condition, then there can only be 1 treatment that works: resection. Moreover, although the role of radiotherapy in osteoradionecrosis is undisputable and at the core of pioneering invaluable refinements to decrease the incidence of osteoradionecrosis,[11,12] the preventive or predisposing role of ablation and reconstruction seems to be largely understated if not overlooked. The improved understanding of the underlying mechanisms in osteoradionecrosis may further warrant a review of the techniques utilized in treating osteoradionecrosis.

Based on this concise introduction, the authors aim at redefining osteoradionecrosis coining a novel term, the osteosarcoradionecrosis, to emphasize the importance of the soft tissue role played in the disease and treatment plan, revising treatment guidelines, taking aggressive approach given that necrosis is death, an irremediable condition, and providing an eye opener on how ablative–reconstructive surgeries may prevent or predispose to osteoradionecrosis.

OSTEOSARCORADIONECROSIS

Osteosarcoradionecrosis is a novel term refers to bicomponent, bone and soft tissue necrosis, following radiotherapy, in which necrosis is death of the tissue, an irreversible condition.

Following irradiation, a cascade of events such as endothelial cell destruction, vascular thrombosis, free radicals release, inflammation, altered osteoblast/osteocast activity, and proliferation of fibroblast into myoblast will ensue to an extent that depends on the intensity of irradiation and the tissue inherent characteristics.[1,5,13,14] It makes sense to speculate that when the bone is injured, other tissues of weaker resistance such as mucosa, skin, and muscles are already damaged, suggesting that the damage to soft tissue could proceed that occurring to the bone. As radiotherapy is applied at the same time, multitissue damage will result in a vicious cycle in which unhealthy skin and mucosa will not support a durable coverage over the bone, leading to soft tissue breakdown and bone exposure, and at the same time the unhealthy bone will not allow the tissue to heal, resulting in sinuses and fistulae. The absence of healthy barrier, mucosa or skin, and the presence of unhealthy bone, may provide a niche for infection, further complicating the situation. Furthermore, the symptoms many of the patients with the previously defined osteoradionecrosis have such as scarring and fibrosis, trismus, atrophy, xerostomia, mucositis, and pain highlight the involvement of the soft tissue. That being said, the chronic wound problem defining osteoradionecrosis is also the result of skin/mucosa necrosis or compromise. The soft tissue, therefore, is at the heart of the problem; this explains the importance of the suggested term "osteosarcoradionecrosis," rather than osteoradionecrosis alone, and allows one to approach the problem from all its aspects as a syndrome following tissue irradiation.

It is essential, however, to avoid liberal use of necrosis. Necrosis should only refer to tissue death,[15] which is irreversible and can only be managed by radical excision. The strict application of necrosis as a term in osteoradionecrosis will give rise the problem of what the condition in which the tissue is undergoing necrosis should be called?

The authors' best answer to this question is dividing the changes following irradiation into 2 major phases that may not be chronologically dependent on each other: the reversible damage phase and the necrosis, irreversible damage, phase. It is important to avoid stressing any chronologic relationship between these 2 phases because radiotherapy-induced damage, which begins with the delivery of radiotherapy, may vary in intensity and extent depending on tissue target, tissue tolerance, and preexisting conditions such as previous surgeries, explaining why some tissue may present with necrosis while irreversible damage could be the situation in some other tissue. The tissue in the reversible phase may reach a statuesque with lifelong risk of osteosarcoradionecrosis, or it becomes irreversibly damaged. The transformation process of phase 1 to 2 can be to a certain extent manipulated by some drugs such as pentoxifylline, tocopherol, clodronate, or steroids.[1,2,6,7]

The authors suggest that the reversible phase may correlate with the prefibrotic phase and the constitutive organized phase,[1,6,7] and it starts with the delivery of radiotherapy and ends once signs of bone and soft tissue necrosis develop clinically, on radiograph, or on histologic examination. The reversible phase could be thus asymptomatic or marked with clinical, radiographic, or histologic signs and symptoms that are not limited to bone inflammation, yet not compatible with necrosis.[1,16,17] The necrosis phase, on the other hand, may correlate with the late fibroatrophoic phase and is marked clinically by: nonhealing wound with bone exposure, fistula, and chronic discharge, and pathologic fractures, which require adequate resection of the necrotic tissue. Necrosis on radiograph such as mixed radio-opaque radiolucent lesion, with the radiolucent areas representing bone destruction, and that spotted by radionuclide bone scanning or on histologic examination in the absence of clinical symptoms will confirm phase 2[1,16,17] but may not warrant immediate surgical intervention, in the authors' opinion.

REFINED TREATMENT PLAN BASED ON THE 2-PHASE CLASSIFICATION

The proposed 2-phase classification may revolutionize how one treats oteosarcoradionecrosis. Although the authors aim not to provide new therapies, they are keen on setting clear guidelines based on the refined understanding available today and the classification proposed in this article.

Based on the successful increased application of medical treatment in early stages/limited and mild forms of osteoradionecrosis, the authors think that the tissue in the reversible phase may benefit from pharmacologic, tissue-rehabilitative, and tissue-regenerative therapies.[1,6,7,18,19] However, the role of hyper baric oxygen therapy could be controversial.[1,19] The goal is to reverse the damage or slow down the transformation process into irreversible necrosis with better control of symptoms. Timing of administration is yet to be defined, but the authors see no contraindications for starting this treatment while the patient is on radiotherapy, and definitely around the time the patient is going to receive any surgical intervention that carries the risk of damaging tissue circulation such as tooth extraction and debridement. To make this approach cost-effective and practical, there could be a need to develop a patient's profile for high-risk osteosarcoradionecrosis based on the institute's own data in collaboration with all disciplines involved such as oncologist, ablative surgeons, and reconstructive surgeon.

On the other hand, osteosarcoradionecrosis, the irreversible phase, should only be treated with resection and reconstruction. Whether the patient presents with a drastic clinical picture of fistula, pathologic fracture and malocclusion, and trismus or simple bone exposure, resection and reconstruction are now considered the treatment of choice. Hyperbaric oxygen therapy and medical treatment have no role here in curing the necrosis,

but may still be indicated as prophylactic treatment should the patient need future surgical treatments.[1,18,19] Free flap reconstruction is the authors' gold standard,[20,21] because reconstruction done this way brings healthy, fresh tissue of regenerative abilities to the area and prohibits further damage to the surrounding tissue when loco-regional flaps are planned, taking into consideration that this tissue could be in an reversible phase or may not be available due to fibrosis and scarring. It is also important to rule out malignancy preoperatively using MRI or computed tomography (CT) scan and postoperatively using histologic examinations[22] (**Fig. 1**).

Is there a role for debridement and sequestroctomy? The osteosarcoradionecrosis could be limited in extent. For instance, intraoral bone exposure measuring 1 to 2 cm with grossly intact skin tempts debridement and direct repair or coverage with local flap. It may sound aggressive to propose resection and free flap reconstruction for this small defect. However, a review of the authors' data from more than 60 cases of osteoradionecrosis treated with resection and free flap reconstruction revealed that although almost all those cases received a series of local debridement, resolution was far from being attainable, with all those cases progressing into a fully blown osteoradionecrosis. This is because, local debridement is an insult in itself that could either amplify or add to the changes induced by radiotherapy or escalate the transformation into the irreversible phase, resulting in bigger defect and unsolved bigger problem. The authors are now, therefore, considering an aggressive approach from the beginning, adequate resection of all necrotic tissue, then bone and soft tissue reconstruction to end the problem once and for all. The low relapse rate the authors' recent findings and previously published data have shown[20-23] may support the notion that early aggressive treatment, which ends patient's suffering and enhances their quality of life, has a minimal risk of recurrence of osteosarcoradionecrosis.

AN EYE OPENER ON THE POSSIBLE ROLE OF RECONSTRUCTION AND ABLATION IN OSTEOSARCORADIONECROSIS OF THE MANDIBLE

Ablative surgery may increase the risk of osteosarcoradionecrosis or predispose to its development, especially, in ablation of advanced tumors.[1,2] The need to achieve total resection of advanced tongue, mouth floor, lower gum and trigone tumors with adequate free margins may necessitate wider excision compromising the circulation of the mandible.[24] In these tumors, it is not uncommon

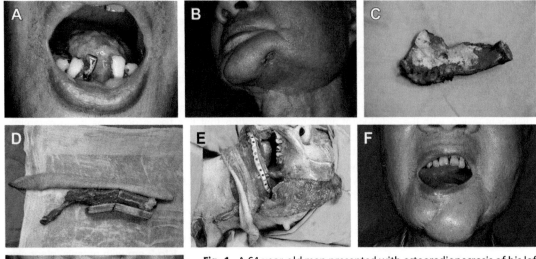

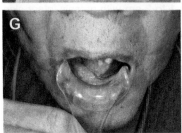

Fig. 1. A 64-year-old man presented with osteoradionecrosis of his left mandible in 2013. He had left tongue cancer; T2N0M0, treated with hemiglossectomy, anterolateral thigh flap reconstruction and postoperative radiotherapy in 2001. (*A*) Tongue reconstruction with an anterolateral thigh flap, appearance in 2005. (*B*) Osteosarcoradionecrosis of the left mandible with persistent purulent discharge from submental region in 2013. (*C*) Resection of necrotic bone and soft tissue. (*D, E*) Segmental mandibular and intraoral lining defects reconstructed with a reconstruction palte and 2-strut fibula osteoseptocutaneous flap. (*F, G*) Post fibula osteoseptocutaneous flap reconstruction at 1-year follow-up.

to perform mandibulotomy as well as marginal mandibulectomy. And in some cases, the mandibular segment that received marginal mandibulectomy is completely stripped of its soft tissue attachment. Marginal mandibulectomy when combined with mandibulotomy will increase the risk of bone necrosis by 70%,[24] and when the bone is further denuded off of its soft tissue cover, the risk could be even higher (**Fig. 2**).

Although it is always important to advise against destructive ablation, it remains impractical, as complete tumor resection may not allow conservative resection. Therefore, it is the responsibility of the reconstructive surgeon to foresee the risk of osteosarcoradionecrosis and revise the reconstructive plan accordingly.

The authors have refined their approach to these challenges utilizing 1 of the following reconstructive options: reconstruction plate only, vascualrized onlay graft, complete resection and reconstruction with reconstruction plate and either a soft tissue flap or vascualrized bone flap, and soft tissue coverage in oversize, overvolume flap.

When mandibulotomy and marginal mandibulectomy have been performed, and the mandible is completely stripped of its soft tissue, the authors may suggest to convert the marginal mandibulectomy into segmental mandibulectomy and reconstruct the bone with either fibula osteoseptocutaneous flap or soft tissue flap depending on patient's functional needs, lesion prognosis, and characteristics of the segmental defect, and taking into account the possible tradeoffs associated with reconstructive techniques.[25]

Alternatively, a vascularized onlay graft such as the fibula osteoseptocutaneous flap can be used for "ike-with-like reconstruction and 1-stage rehabilitation of the mandibile, a technique similar to using the fibula for the salvage of pathologic fractures of long bones.[26] This option may also bring a new source of vascualrization to the bone, which is the bone marrow of the vascualrized fibula flap. If the patient is not a good candidate for such a procedure, a large soft tissue flap can be used to fill the defect of the marginal mandibulectomy and protect the bone from radiotherapy. The need for a reconstruction plate should be assessed based on the height of the mandible postmarginal mandibulectomy and the length of the marginal defect (**Fig. 3**). Alternatively, a reconstructive plate alone can be used, given that adequate soft tissue coverage is left after resection in laterally placed marginal mandibulectomies.

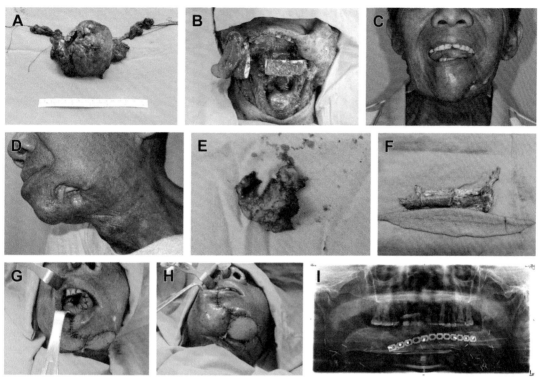

Fig. 2. 45-year-old man presented with osteosarcoradionecrosis of his left mandible. His history was significant for left tongue squamous cell carcinoma cancer T4aN2b, treated by totoal glossectomy, and marginal mandibulectomy and midline mandibulotomy, anterolateral thigh flap, and radiotherapy. (*A*) Total glossectomy and marginal madnibulectomy in 2014. (*B*) Combined mandibulotomy and marginal mandibulectomy, the marginal mandibular segment is denuded off the soft tissue in 2014. (*C*) An anterolateral thigh flap for reconstruction of total tongue and marginal mandibular defect in 2014. (*D*) Bone exposure with orocutaneous fistula in March 2015. (*E, F*) Markings for the fibula osteoseptocutaneous flap and the flap after ostetomies in September 2015. (*G, H*) Appearance at the end of surgery in September 2015. (*I*) Recent panorex showing the mandible necrosis free after definite resection and fibula osteoseptocutaneous flap reconstruction.

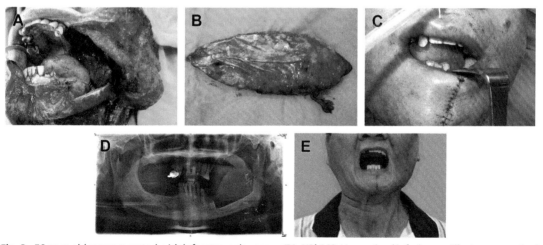

Fig. 3. 56-year-old man presented with left retromolar cancer T4aN2bM0. He received inferior maxillectomy, marginal madnibulectomy, and anterolateral thigh flap reconstruction after radiotherapy was delivered. (*A*) The defect after resection of retromolar cancer, in 2014. It involved inferior maxillectomy, buccal defect, and marginal mandibulectomy; note the adequate height of the residual mandible. (*B*) An anterolateral thigh flap was harvested for defect reconstruction and restoration of the mandible contour. (*C*) Appearance after at the end of the reconstructive surgery. (*D*) Follow-up panorex: no fracture or suspected osteoradionecrosis. (*E*) Appearance in 2016: good contour.

The soft tissue utilized to provide bone protection or bone defect obliteration could be a deepithelialized skin or viable muscle or a combination of both in oversize and overvolume flap. It is important to mention, however, that this approach needs particular planning and consideration in flap design and inset. Otherwise, trying to utilize whatever tissue is redundant after inset may force the surgeon to use unreliable part of the flap, provide inadequate coverage, or even compromise the reconstruction by stretching the flap too thin to fulfill many goals not fully addressed in planning and design, resulting in complications rather than solutions.

SUMMARY

Osteosarcoradionecrosis is a novel term that addresses the soft tissue role in osteoradionecrosis. The 2-phase classification proposed may provide simplified and straightforward treatment guideline to osteosarcoradionecrosis of the head and neck. The authors' refined reconstructive approach to the marginal mandibulectomy defect may help decrease complications following radiotherapy.

REFERENCES

1. Chrcanovic BR, Reher P, Sousa AA, et al. Osteoradionecrosis of the jaws–a current overview–part 1: physiopathology and risk and predisposing factors. Oral Maxillofac Surg 2010;14(1):3–16.

2. Lambade PN, Lambade D, Goel M. Osteoradionecrosis of the mandible: a review. Oral Maxillofac Surg 2013;17(4):243–9.

3. Meyer I. Infectious diseases of the jaws. J Oral Surg 1970;28:17–26.

4. Marx RE. Osteoradionecrosis: a new concept of its pathophysiology. J Oral Maxillofac Surg 1983;41:283–8.

5. Delanian S, Lefaix JL. The radiation-induced fibroatrophic process: therapeutic perspective via the antioxidant pathway. Radiother Oncol 2004;73:119–31.

6. Delanian S, Depondt J, Lefaix JL. Major healing of refractory mandible osteoradionecrosis after treatment combining pentoxifylline and tocopherol: a phase II trial. Head Neck 2005;27:114–23.

7. Epstein JB, Wong FLW, Stevenson-Moore P. Osteoradionecrosis: clinical experience and a proposal for classification. J Oral Maxillofac Surg 1987;45(2):104–10.

8. Schwartz HC, Kagan AR. Osteoradionecrosis of the mandible: scientific basis for clinical staging. Am J Clin Oncol 2002;25(2):168–71.

9. Marx RE, Ehler WJ, Tayapongsak P, et al. Relationship of oxygen dose to angiogenesis induction in irradiated tissue. Am J Surg 1990;160(5):519–24.

10. Jansma J, Vissink A, Spijkervet FKL, et al. Protocol for the prevention and treatment of oral sequelae resulting from head and neck radiation therapy. Cancer 1992;70:2171–80.

11. Ahmed M, Hansen VN, Harrington KJ, et al. Reducing the risk of xerostomia and mandibular osteoradionecrosis: the potential benefits of intensity modulated radiotherapy in advanced oral cavity carcinoma. Med Dosim 2009;34(3):217–24.

12. Nguyen NP, Vock J, Chi A, et al. Effectiveness of intensity-modulated and image-guided radiotherapy to spare the mandible from excessive radiation. Oral Oncol 2012;48(7):653–7.

13. Assael LA. New foundations in understanding osteonecrosis of the jaws. J Oral Maxillofac Surg 2004;62:125–6.

14. Al-Nawas B, Duschner H, Grötz KA. Early cellular alterations in bone after radiation therapy and its relation to osteoradionecrosis. J Oral Maxillofac Surg 2004;62:1045.

15. Available at: www.merriam-webster.com/medical/necrosis.

16. Store G, Boysen M. Mandibular osteoradionecrosis: clinical behaviour and diagnostic aspects. Clin Otolaryngol Allied Sci 2000;25:378–84.

17. Reuther T, Schuster T, Mende U, et al. Osteoradionecrosis of the jaws as a side effect of radiotherapy of head and neck tumour patients—a report of a thirty-year retrospective review. Int J Oral Maxillofac Surg 2003;32:289–95.

18. Lyons A, Osher J, Warner E, et al. Osteoradionecrosis—a review of current concepts in defining the extent of the disease and a new classification proposal. Br J Oral Maxillofac Surg 2014;52(5):392–5.

19. D'Souza J, Lowe D, Rogers SN. Changing trends and the role of medical management on the outcome of patients treated for osteoradionecrosis of the mandible: experience from a regional head and neck unit. Br J Oral Maxillofac Surg 2014;52(4):356–62.

20. Santamaria E, Wei FC, Chen HC. Fibula osteoseptocutaneous flap for reconstruction of osteoradionecrosis of the mandible. Plast Reconstr Surg 1998;101(4):921–9.

21. Coskunfirat OK, Wei FC, Huang WC, et al. Microvascular free tissue transfer for treatment of osteoradionecrosis of the maxilla. Plast Reconstr Surg 2005;115(1):54–60.

22. Hao SP, Chen HC, Wei FC, et al. Systematic management of osteoradionecrosis in the head and neck. Laryngoscope 1999;109(8):1324–7 [discussion: 1327–8].

23. Celik N, Wei FC, Chen HC, et al. Osteoradionecrosis of the mandible after oromandibular cancer surgery. Plast Reconstr Surg 2002;109(6):1875–81.

24. Wang CC, Cheng MH, Hao SP, et al. Osteoradio-necrosis with combined mandibulotomy and marginal mandibulectomy. Laryngoscope 2005;115(11):1963–7.

25. Wei FC, Celik N, Yang WG, et al. Complications after reconstruction by plate and soft-tissue free flap in composite mandibular defects and secondary salvage reconstruction with osteocutaneous flap. Plast Reconstr Surg 2003;112(1):37–42.

26. Friedrich JB, Moran SL, Bishop AT, et al. Vascular-ized fibula flap onlay for salvage of pathologic frac-ture of the long bones. Plast Reconstr Surg 2008; 121(6):2001–9.

Index

Note: Page numbers of article titles are in **boldface** type.

Clin Plastic Surg 43 (2016) 761–764
http://dx.doi.org/10.1016/S0094-1298(16)30104-3
0094-1298/16/$ – see front matter

UNITED STATES POSTAL SERVICE®

Statement of Ownership, Management, and Circulation
(All Periodicals Publications Except Requester Publications)

1. Publication Title	2. Publication Number	3. Filing Date
CLINICS IN PLASTIC SURGERY	006 – 530	9/18/2016

4. Issue Frequency	5. Number of Issues Published Annually	6. Annual Subscription Price
JAN, APR, JUL, OCT	4	$466.00

7. Complete Mailing Address of Known Office of Publication (Not printer) (Street, city, county, state, and ZIP+4®)

ELSEVIER INC.
360 PARK AVENUE SOUTH
NEW YORK, NY 10010-1710

Contact Person
STEPHEN R. BUSHING

Telephone (Include area code)
215-239-3688

8. Complete Mailing Address of Headquarters or General Business Office of Publisher (Not printer)

ELSEVIER INC.
360 PARK AVENUE SOUTH
NEW YORK, NY 10010-1710

9. Full Names and Complete Mailing Addresses of Publisher, Editor, and Managing Editor (Do not leave blank)

Publisher (Name and complete mailing address)

LINDA BELFUS, ELSEVIER INC.
1600 JOHN F KENNEDY BLVD. SUITE 1800
PHILADELPHIA, PA 19103-2899

Editor (Name and complete mailing address)

JESSICA McCOOL, ELSEVIER INC.
1600 JOHN F KENNEDY BLVD. SUITE 1800
PHILADELPHIA, PA 19103-2899

Managing Editor (Name and complete mailing address)

BARBARA COHEN-KLIGERMAN, ELSEVIER INC.
1600 JOHN F KENNEDY BLVD. SUITE 1800
PHILADELPHIA, PA 19103-2899

10. Owner (Do not leave blank. If the publication is owned by a corporation, give the name and address of the corporation immediately followed by the names and addresses of all stockholders owning or holding 1 percent or more of the total amount of stock. If not owned by a corporation, give the names and addresses of the individual owners. If owned by a partnership or other unincorporated firm, give its name and address as well as those of each individual owner. If the publication is published by a nonprofit organization, give its name and address.)

Full Name	Complete Mailing Address
WHOLLY OWNED SUBSIDIARY OF REED/ELSEVIER, US HOLDINGS	1600 JOHN F KENNEDY BLVD. SUITE 1800 PHILADELPHIA, PA 19 03-2899

11. Known Bondholders, Mortgagees, and Other Security Holders Owning or Holding 1 Percent or More of Total Amount of Bonds, Mortgages, or Other Securities. If none, check box ▸ ☐ None

Full Name	Complete Mailing Address
N/A	

12. Tax Status (For completion by nonprofit organizations authorized to mail at nonprofit rates) (Check one)
The purpose, function, and nonprofit status of this organization and the exempt status for federal income tax purposes:
☐ Has Not Changed During Preceding 12 Months
☐ Has Changed During Preceding 12 Months (Publisher must submit explanation of change with this statement)

13. Publication Title	14. Issue Date for Circulation Data Below
CLINICS IN PLASTIC SURGERY	JULY 2016

15. Extent and Nature of Circulation			Average No. Copies Each Issue During Preceding 12 Months	No. Copies of Single Issue Published Nearest to Filing Date
a. Total Number of Copies (Net press run)			584	745
b. Paid Circulation (By Mail and Outside the Mail)	(1)	Mailed Outside-County Paid Subscriptions Stated on PS Form 3541 (Include paid distribution above nominal rate, advertiser's proof copies, and exchange copies)	221	279
	(2)	Mailed In-County Paid Subscriptions Stated on PS Form 3541 (Include paid distribution above nominal rate, advertiser's proof copies, and exchange copies)	0	0
	(3)	Paid Distribution Outside the Mails Including Sales Through Dealers and Carriers, Street Vendors, Counter Sales, and Other Paid Distribution Outside USPS®	129	173
	(4)	Paid Distribution by Other Classes of Mail Through the USPS (e.g., First-Class Mail®)	0	0
c. Total Paid Distribution (Sum of 15b (1), (2), (3), and (4))			350	452
d. Free or Nominal Rate Distribution (By Mail and Outside the Mail)	(1)	Free or Nominal Rate Outside-County Copies Included on PS Form 3541	61	93
	(2)	Free or Nominal Rate In-County Copies Included on PS Form 3541	0	0
	(3)	Free or Nominal Rate Copies Mailed at Other Classes Through the USPS (e.g., First-Class Mail)	0	0
	(4)	Free or Nominal Rate Distribution Outside the Mail (Carriers or other means)	0	0
e. Total Free or Nominal Rate Distribution (Sum of 15d (1), (2), (3) and (4))			61	93
f. Total Distribution (Sum of 15c and 15e)			411	545
g. Copies not Distributed (See Instructions to Publishers #4 (page #3))			173	200
h. Total (Sum of 15f and g)			584	745
i. Percent Paid (15c divided by 15f times 100)			85%	83%

* If you are claiming electronic copies, go to line 16 on page 3. If you are not claiming electronic copies, skip to line 17 on page 3.

16. Electronic Copy Circulation	Average No. Copies Each Issue During Preceding 12 Months	No. Copies of Single Issue Published Nearest to Filing Date
a. Paid Electronic Copies	0	0
b. Total Paid Print Copies (Line 15c) + Paid Electronic Copies (Line 16a)	350	452
c. Total Print Distribution (Line 15f) + Paid Electronic Copies (Line 16a)	411	545
d. Percent Paid (Both Print & Electronic Copies) (16b divided by 16c × 100)	85%	83%

☒ I certify that 50% of all my distributed copies (electronic and print) are paid above a nominal price.

17. Publication of Statement of Ownership

☒ If the publication is a general publication, publication of this statement is required. Will be printed ☐ Publication not required.
in the OCTOBER 2016 issue of this publication.

18. Signature and Title of Editor, Publisher, Business Manager, or Owner

STEPHEN R. BUSHING - INVENTORY DISTRIBUTION CONTROL MANAGER

Date 9/18/2016

I certify that all information furnished on this form is true and complete. I understand that anyone who furnishes false or misleading information on this form or who omits material or information requested on the form may be subject to criminal sanctions (including fines and imprisonment) and/or civil sanctions (including civil penalties).

PS Form 3526, July 2014 (Page 3 of 4) PRIVACY NOTICE: See our privacy policy on www.usps.com.

PS Form 3526, July 2014 (Page 1 of 4 (see instructions page 4)) PSN: 7530-01-000-9931 PRIVACY NOTICE: See our privacy policy on www.usps.com.

Moving?

Make sure your subscription moves with you!

To notify us of your new address, find your **Clinics Account Number** (located on your mailing label above your name), and contact customer service at:

Email: journalscustomerservice-usa@elsevier.com

800-654-2452 (subscribers in the U.S. & Canada)
314-447-8871 (subscribers outside of the U.S. & Canada)

Fax number: 314-447-8029

Elsevier Health Sciences Division
Subscription Customer Service
3251 Riverport Lane
Maryland Heights, MO 63043

*To ensure uninterrupted delivery of your subscription, please notify us at least 4 weeks in advance of move.

Printed and bound by CPI Group (UK) Ltd, Croydon, CR0 4YY

08/05/2025

01864686-0019